LOW-FODMAP PALEO COOKBOOK

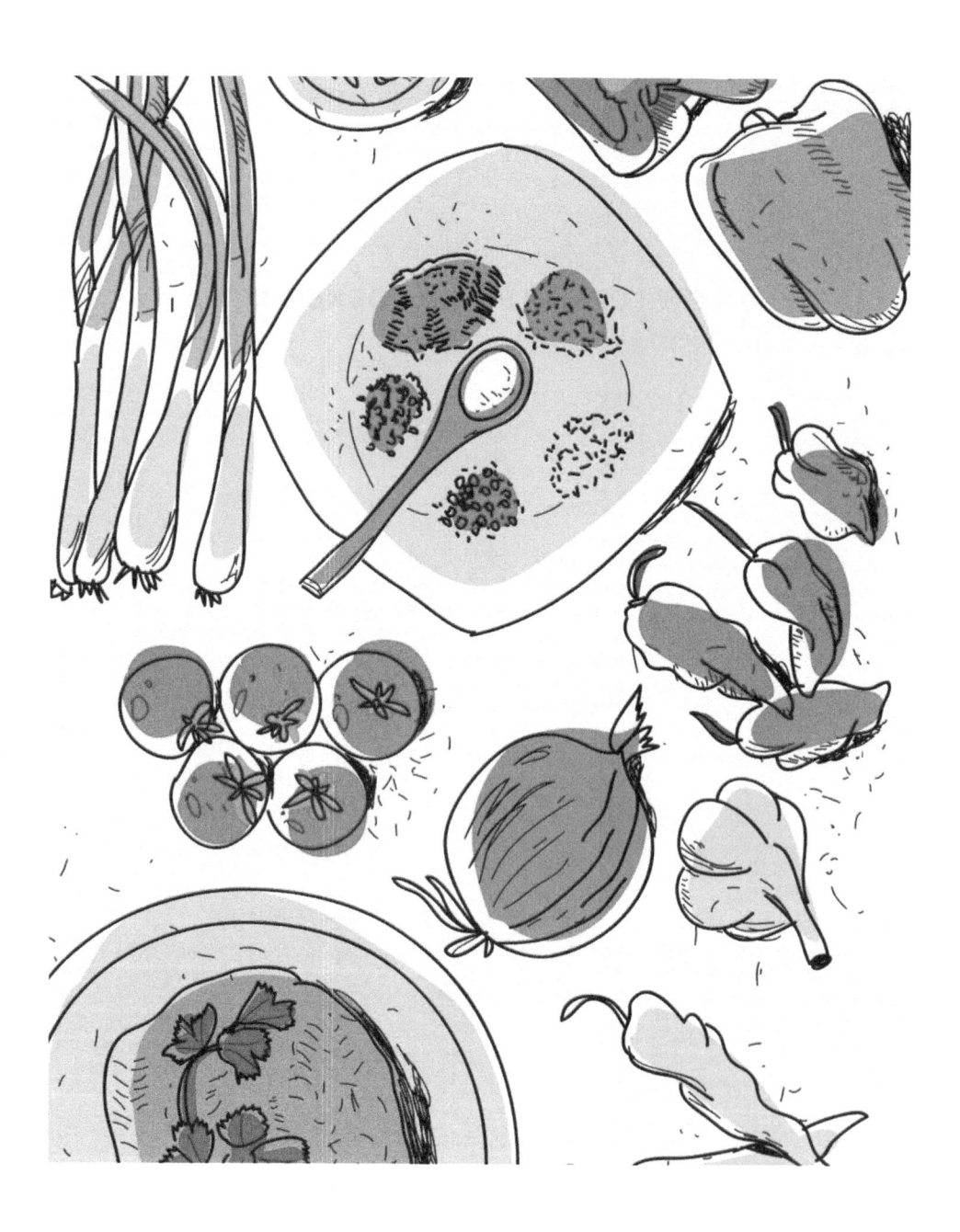

Low-FODMAP Paleo Cookbook

The Revolutionary Diet for Managing IBS, Inflammation and Other Digestive Disorders

Ingrid Morano

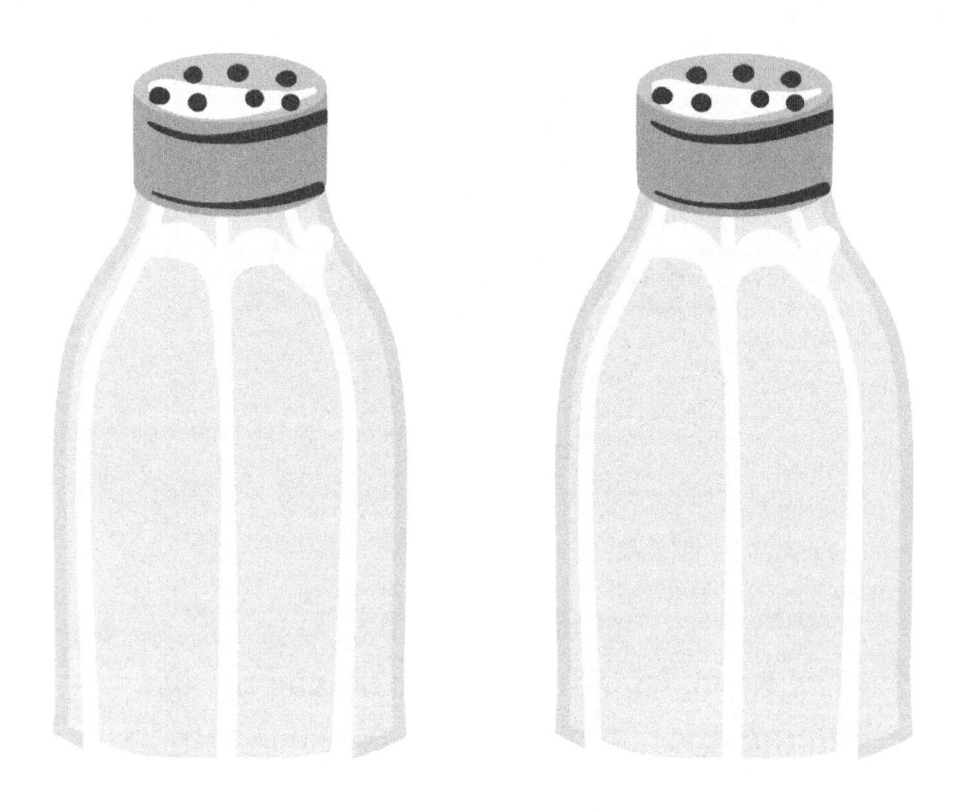

LEGAL NOTICE

Copyright (c) 2019 by Ingrid Morano

All rights are reserved. No portion of this book may be reproduced or duplicated using any form whether mechanical, electronic, or otherwise. No portion of this book may be transmitted, stored in a retrieval database, or otherwise made available in any manner whether public or private unless specific permission is granted by the publisher. Vector illustration credit: vecteezy.com

This book does not offer advice, but merely provides information. The author offers no advice whether medical, financial, legal, or otherwise, nor does the author encourage any person to pursue any specific course of action discussed in this book. This book is not a substitute for professional advice. The reader accepts complete and sole responsibility for the manner in which this book and its contents are used. The publisher and the author will not be held liable for any damages caused.

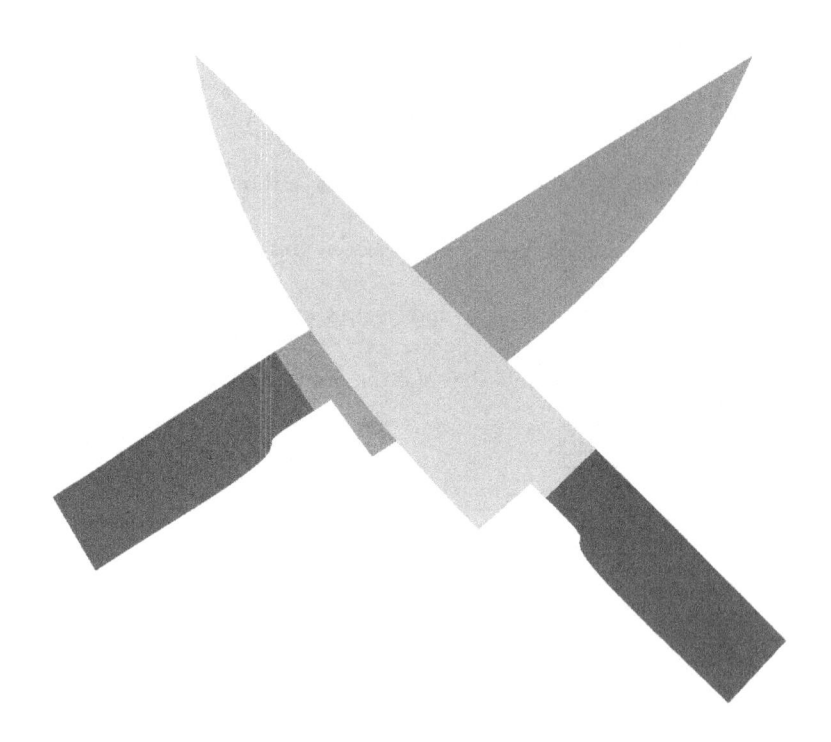

CONTENTS

GOING PALEO THE LOW-FODMAP WAY 9
INTRODUCTION TO PALEO LOW FODMAP DIET 11
BREAKFAST RECIPES 21
LUNCH RECIPES 53
DINNER RECIPES 85
DESSERT RECIPES 117
REFERENCES AND RESOURCES 128
THE "DIRTY DOZEN" AND "CLEAN 15" 131
MEASUREMENT CONVERSION TABLES 133
INDEX 134

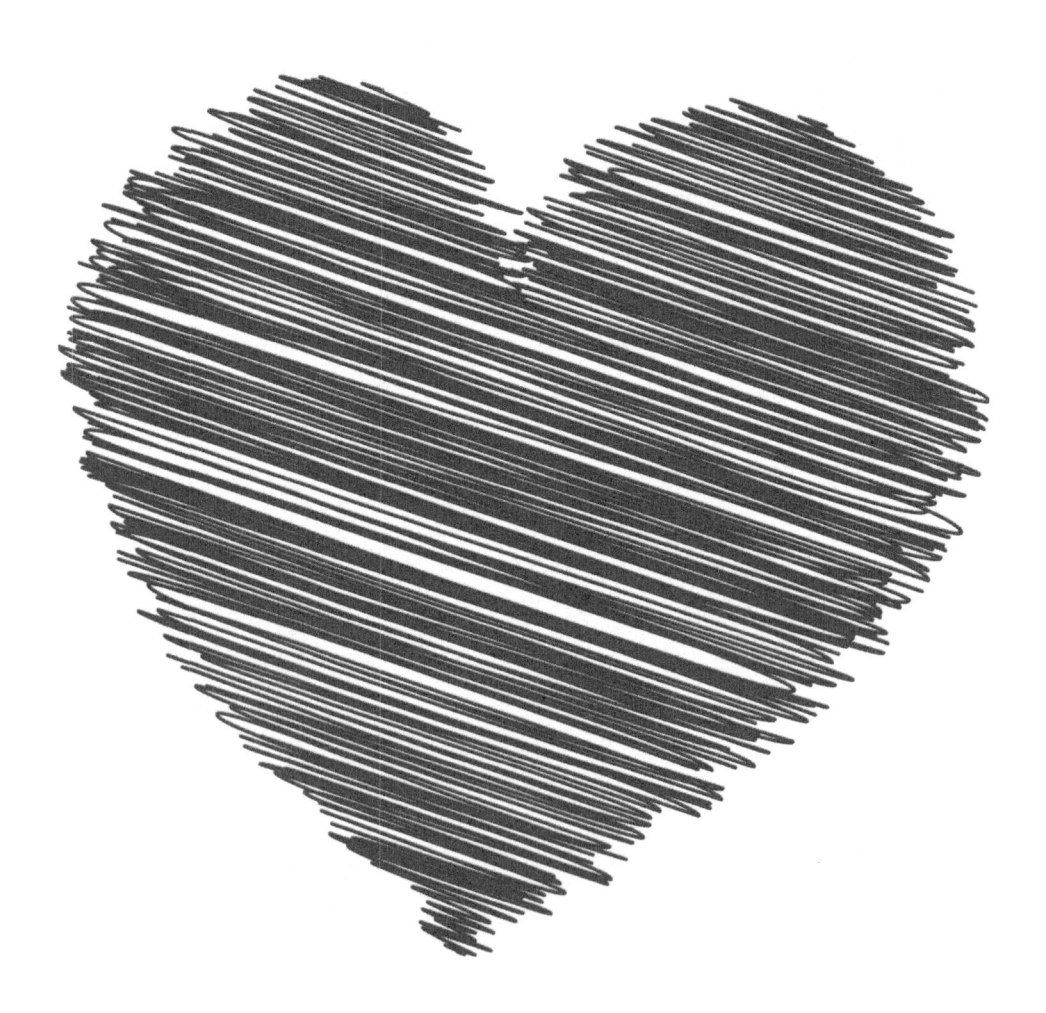

GOING PALEO THE LOW-FODMAP WAY

Food can either heal, help, or harm. When it heals, it's fueling your energy, nourishing your body, and building your strength. When it helps, it's providing the nutrients and sustenance you need to maintain good health. When it harms, it's working against your best interests, and not giving you what you need. Unfortunately, much of the food we eat today is harmful. Decades of processing, stripping out good nutrients, and stuffing in sugar and artificial ingredients have turned what should heal and help us into something that does the opposite.

This is a big reason why people are embracing going Paleo. Based on the theory that our Paleolithic-era ancestors were healthy and not vulnerable to the kinds of health problems we have today, going Paleo is about mimicking their diet. They didn't eat grains or dairy, and they certainly weren't eating anything processed. Instead, they were eating lots of vegetables, meat, certain fruits, nuts, seeds, and certain oils. By returning to this eating lifestyle, many people have discovered the healing and helpful powers of food.

Going Paleo may not be enough, however, if you are like me. I am one of the many people out there with a digestive disorder, and we know all too well the harmful impacts of food. While food doesn't cause a disorder, it does aggravate it, and finding things to eat can seem like a minefield. This stress makes symptoms worse, and it all starts to take a toll. Food can feel like a cage. I know I found myself asking: is it possible to find freedom by being Paleo?

The answer is yes, but first, consider the Low FODMAP diet. Developed at Australia's Monash University, this 3-phase diet is all about simple carbs known as FODMAPs, which are found in high amounts in certain foods like apples, wheat, artificial sweeteners, beans, and so on. If you eat a lot of high FODMAP foods, the small intestine isn't able to break them down properly, and they end up in the large intestine. There, they ferment and cause digestive symptoms like gas, diarrhea, and more. If you have a GI disorder, you are especially vulnerable, and high FODMAPs can wreak havoc on your compromised system. The Low FODMAP diet is about identifying which high FODMAPs you're especially sensitive to, which ones are okay, and reducing your symptoms.

On Phase 1 of the Low FODMAP diet, which lasts around 2-6 weeks, you eliminate high FODMAP foods from your diet. Replace them with low FODMAP alternatives. This gives your body a chance to heal and reset. For me, phase 1 was hard, and I think it is for most people. You are eliminating *a lot* of food, and finding replacements takes time and effort. The meals I made frequently needed to be adjusted, and going out to eat could be tricky. However, once I got into a groove, I started feeling better than I had in years. I started feeling hopeful that this could be my future.

Phase 2 of the Low FODMAP diet is about reintroducing foods back into your diet to see what exactly aggravates your symptoms. This part wasn't especially fun, and it can be stressful for a lot of people. You might be tempted to stay on phase 1 longer, just to keep feeling better, but that puts you at risk for nutritional deficiencies. Phase 1 of the Low FODMAP is designed to be short, and just long enough to get the high FODMAPs out of your system. Don't feel too stressed about phase 2. Most people are only sensitive to a small number of high FODMAP foods, and many of them are not inherently harmful or bad. Remember, because you are also Paleo, you won't add in certain foods like grains, beans, and dairy. According to the principles of being Paleo, these are not healing or helpful.

Once you've added back in Paleo-friendly high FODMAPs, you can now live a very customized Paleo lifestyle. That's phase 3, which is your permanent diet. I've been on mine for a few years now, and it's been the best few years of my life. I feel in control of my digestive disorder, and not the only way around. I know exactly what foods to avoid and which foods to limit, and which foods are perfectly fine. There's no minefield anymore, and no cage.

In this book, you'll learn what you can and can't eat when you're Paleo, and more specifics on how the Low FODMAP diet works. Together, they can be a very effective diet for people with a digestive disorder, whether it's IBS, Crohn's, or SIBO. However, as with any restrictive diet, there are risks. You might change too much too quickly, and become overwhelmed, which prevents your body from healing and resetting properly. The Paleo Low FODMAP diet can also put you at risk for micronutrient deficiencies, which is common with any diet that cuts out entire food groups. It's also common to succumb to disordered eating, which is an obsession with food quality and a diet's rules, leading to stress and health issues. To avoid these risks and live life to the fullest, this book also lays out tips for success.

Do you want your diet to be healing and helpful, or harmful? That's an easy question. *How* to get there, however, might have been the real issue for you. With the Paleo Low FODMAP diet, you can figure out what causes your symptoms and then design a Paleo-based diet that fuels the life you want. You don't have to live in pain and anxiety because of what you eat.

Freedom is possible.
Ingrid Morano

INTRODUCTION TO PALEO LOW FODMAP DIET

What we eat has a huge effect on our health, and if you are dealing with a digestive disorder like IBS or Crohn's, you know more than others how true that is. There are seemingly-countless diets out there claiming to be healthy, so how do you choose? Getting good information is key, and that's what this section is all about. The diet we're talking about is the Paleo Low FODMAP diet, a combination of two popular eating plans. Before we dive in, let's first learn about each one separately, so you have a good foundation. If you are already Paleo or know about the Low FODMAP diet, you can skip the relevant sections and get right to the combo diet.

BEING PALEO

In 2002, Dr. Loren Cordain began exploring eating styles that could push back against processed foods and their health consequences. His research took him way back in time, to the Paleolithic era, and he believed our distant ancestors were actually healthier than we were. Why? Because of what they were eating. They weren't growing grain or dairy, and instead lived on the meat they caught and produce they foraged. They weren't eating sugar, either, except the small amount found in fruit. While a lot of time has passed since humans started eating grains, dairy, and more sugar, Dr. Cordain believed our bodies haven't adjusted fast enough. To get healthier, he claimed we needed to get back to basics.

How Paleo works

Dr. Cordain wrote a book and laid out what it meant to go Paleo. Basically, we needed to eat only what was available to Paleolithic people, so no dairy, grain, and of course, no processed food. 55% of the diet needed to be lean meat and seafood, with 15% from fruit, 15% from veggies, and 15% from seeds and nuts. A lot of people don't follow those exact percentages, but they're definitely a guide.

Unlike a lot of diets, you don't need to count calories when you're Paleo. It's a lifestyle and philosophy for many people. They try to exercise in a way that lines up with what Paleolithic humans might have done, like climbing, hiking, and swimming. Our ancestors also didn't have the stresses of modern life, so many dieters try to get outside, use their phones less, and socialize more. Combined with the diet, this type of life can significantly improve a person's health.

What you can eat

Going Paleo isn't too complicated, as long as you remember that quality is important, and if you're in doubt, ask yourself, "Would a Paleolithic person have access to this?"

Here's what you are allowed to eat:

High-quality meat + seafood

This means grass-fed beef without antibiotics and pasture-raised chickens. Other organic meat, like lamb, goat, veal, bison, and so on are also on the table. As for seafood, anything that's wild-caught is fair game, including clams, salmon, shrimp, tuna, and so on.

Eggs

Organic is the way to go.

Fruit

Most fruit is allowed when you're Paleo, though you should remember that Paleolithics weren't growing orchards or anything. Their fruit would also have been very different and contained less sugar. Berries are the best choice. Fruits like apples, grapes, mangoes, oranges, peaches, pineapple, and so on should be eaten in moderation if weight loss is your goal.

Vegetables

Eat vegetables freely and frequently when you're Paleo. The only ones you should watch your intake of are starchy ones like sweet potatoes and squash, just because they don't have quite as much nutrition by volume.

Nuts + seeds

Paleolithics would have eaten nuts and seeds quite often. They are important for their fat content and they make you feel satisfied. All nuts and seeds (almonds, cashews, macadamia nuts, sunflower seeds, etc) are acceptable.

Oils + fats

There's some debate about whether you should cook with olive oil or just eat it raw. You can definitely cook with clarified butter (ghee) or animal fat, like tallow or duck fat. You can also eat avocado oil, coconut oil, and macadamia nut oil. Whether or not you cook with them is up to you.

Drinks

Not surprisingly, pretty much all drinks wouldn't been around for Paleolithic people. You are limited to water, herbal tea, and sometimes 100% fruit juice.

Note: There are certain foods in the gray area, and lots of people following a Paleo lifestyle do include them. Over time, there's also been changes and adjustments based on what Paleo experts are learning about the past, and on what allows the lifestyle to be sustainable. It's up to you to develop what works best for you. Some gray-area foods include:

- Vinegars (apple cider, balsamic)
- Buttermilk
- Mascarpone cheese
- Bittersweet chocolate
- Potato flour
- Homemade almond milk (just water and almonds)
- Goat's milk
- Sesame seed oil
- Raw honey
- Maple syrup
- Whiskey
- Black coffee

What you can't eat

If it isn't on that list above, you most likely can't eat it if you're going Paleo. Foods include:

- *All grain/legumes/beans* - wheat, rice, quinoa, pasta, barley, soy, tofu, beans, chickpeas
- *All dairy* - cheese, butter, milk, yogurt
- *All sweeteners* - natural (i.e. sugar, stevia) and artificial (i.e. splenda)
- *Processed meat* - deli ham, spam, hot dogs, roast beef
- *Certain oils/salad dressings* - canola oil, bottled salad dressings
- *Processed snack food*- granola bars, candy, chips
- *Certain drinks* - energy drinks, soda, alcohol

WHAT ARE FODMAPS?

First off, what *are* FODMAPs exactly? It's shorthand for a mouthful of science words: fermentable oligosaccharides, disaccharides, monosaccharides, and polyols. To simplify, these are short-chain, simple carbs. They're found in certain foods like veggies, dairy, grain, beans, sweeteners, and fruit. They're not as plentiful in meat, seafood, fats, and oils. Why do FODMAPs matter? They have a certain effect on the body.

FODMAPs aren't inherently bad for you. If they were, we wouldn't be able to eat any veggies, fruit, beans, grain, etc. However, if you eat too many FODMAPs, it is harder for the small intestine (which absorbs most nutrients) to break them down. If not properly absorbed, FODMAPs move to the large intestine, which isn't able to absorb many nutrients. The FODMAPs hang out there, interacting with bacteria, and they start to ferment. This triggers symptoms like gas, and the FODMAPs start pulling water into the intestinal tract, causing issues like diarrhea. If not addressed, more serious health problems can occur.

FODMAPs are especially bothersome if you have a digestive disorder. You are more sensitive to the symptoms of fermentation in the large intestine. Here are some of the digestive disorders that too many FODMAPs can aggravate:

IBS (IRRITABLE BOWEL SYNDROME)

IBS manifests in the large intestine and causes symptoms like stomach pain, bloating, gas, constipation, and diarrhea. More serious problems can occur, as well, like weight loss, constant stomach pain, and frequent diarrhea in the middle of the night. It's a chronic disease, but can be managed to the point where life is normal. Experts aren't sure what causes IBS, but it could be an issue with muscle contractions, inflammation, or changes in gut bacteria. FODMAPs can aggravate the disease, but they don't cause IBS.

CROHN'S DISEASE

Unlike IBS, Crohn's tends to target the small intestine, though it can extend to any part of the digestive tract. It manifests as inflammation, and while symptoms often start out mild, they worsen as time goes on. Symptoms include stomach pain, anemia, diarrhea, fatigue, nausea, and so on. Stress tends to aggravate this chronic disease, as well as certain foods, like those with high FODMAPs. Genetics may play a role in who gets Crohn's, though it could also be an autoimmune condition. Doctors aren't sure. When managed, someone with Crohn's can go into remission for weeks or even years.

SIBO (SMALL INTESTINAL BACTERIAL OVERGROWTH)

In a healthy person, the small bowel gets rid of excess bacteria. However, when that doesn't happen, the bacteria builds up and eventually starts consuming the nutrition the body needs. This can cause malnutrition. Symptoms include stomach cramps, diarrhea, fatigue, nausea, and other digestive issues. People with SIBO report other problems, too, like depression, anxiety, joint pain, and asthma. Certain foods can aggravate symptoms. Causes of SIBO vary and include genetics, inflamed digestive tract, slow bowels, a poor diet, and an autoimmune reaction.

THE LOW FODMAP DIET

Now that you know more about FODMAPs and why they can be a problem, let's get into the Low FODMAP diet. It was developed by researchers and experts at Monash University in Australia. They looked at IBS, specifically, and collected data on the amount of FODMAPs in a huge variety of food. With this information, they developed the three phases of the Low FODMAP diet:

Phase 1: Elimination

This is the strictest phase of the diet. It's meant to provide a reset for your body, so you need to eliminate *all* foods with the highest FODMAPs. This phase is meant to be short-term, because lots of high FODMAP foods are nutritionally-valuable, but for this phase, you don't know what is aggravating your symptoms. Your body needs a blank slate. Since we're going to be talking about a Paleo-style Low FODMAP diet soon, we won't list all the foods you need to eliminate now, but they include certain meat, certain vegetables, certain beverages, and so on. To balance your diet, you will need to be sure to replace high FODMAPs with low FODMAPs, so you aren't starving yourself. Most doctors recommend staying on this phase for just 2-6 weeks.

Phase 2: Reintroduction

After 2-6 weeks, your symptoms should be very mild or reduced entirely. Now it's time to reintroduce high FODMAPs and identify which specific ones are aggravating. You add groups in one at a time, and if your body doesn't react negatively to them, they can stay in your diet. If they do cause problems, you will know you should avoid them. Depending on the severity of the aggravation, you can try to reduce the volume of a specific food and see if things improve. Oftentimes, it's the *amount* of a certain food, and not the food itself, that is a problem. Sometimes, you might learn that even a small amount aggravates you, so you will just have to avoid it completely. This phase takes as long as you need it to.

Phase 3: Maintenance

This is essentially your long-term diet. Based on what you learned in phase 2 about which high FODMAPs are okay or not, you just live your life eating foods that don't aggravate your symptoms. Be aware of what you eat and how much of things you eat, so if your symptoms start up again, you can look back and identify what might have been the problem.

The Paleo Low FODMAP diet

It's time to combine the two diets we just discussed. When you go Paleo, you eliminate certain foods, and some of these cross over to the Low FODMAP diet and phase 1, but because it isn't Paleo, you would never reintroduce it. There are also certain foods you would usually be allowed to eat during phase 1 that are off the table permanently because of the Paleo rules. Eventually, you basically just become Paleo, because Low FODMAP is more of a protocol than a "diet," per say. What makes your Paleo lifestyle different is that you pay closer attention to how certain foods affect your body and GI disorder symptoms.

To keep things easy for you, here's two food lists for what you eliminate on phase 1 and what you're allowed to eat during all three phases of the Paleo Low FODMAP diet.

> **Note: If you've been Paleo for a while, certain foods below would already be missing from your diet, but in case you're new to Paleo, we're including those and marking them as eliminated forever.**

What you can't eat on Paleo Low FODMAP Phase 1:

Certain meat

- Chorizo (would never reintroduce)
- Sausage (would never reintroduce)

Certain vegetables

- Artichoke
- Asparagus
- Beets
- Broccoli
- Brussels sprouts
- Cabbage
- Cauliflower
- Fennel
- Garlic
- Leeks
- Mushrooms
- Okra
- Onion
- Pickled vegetables
- Scallions
- Shallots
- Snow peas
- Sun-dried tomatoes

Certain fruit

- Apples
- Apricots
- Avocado
- Blackberries
- Cherries
- Dates
- Dried pineapple
- Figs
- Grapefruit
- Guava
- Mango
- Nectarines
- Peaches
- Pears
- Plums
- Pomegranates
- Prunes
- Raisins
- Watermelon

All dairy (would never reintroduce)

- Animal milk
- Cheese
- Heavy cream
- Ice cream/gelato/custard
- Kefir
- Sour cream
- Yogurt

All beans (would never reintroduce)

- Black
- Black-eyed peas
- Broad
- Butter
- Haricot
- Kidney
- Lima
- Mung
- Soy
- Split

All grain (would never reintroduce)

- Almond meal
- Amaranth flour
- Barley
- Couscous
- Oats
- Rye
- Semolina
- Spelt
- Wheat

Certain nuts

- Cashews
- Pistachios

All sweeteners + condiments (would never reintroduce)

- Agave
- All sweeteners ending in "-tol"
- Fruit jam
- High-fructose corn syrup
- Honey (maybe reintroduce, depending on your opinion of raw honey as "Paleo")
- Hummus
- Isomalt
- Molasses
- Pesto
- Relish
- Tahini

Certain drinks

- Beer (would not reintroduce)
- Black tea (would not reintroduce)
- Chamomile tea
- Coconut water (would not reintroduce)
- Fennel tea
- Fruit juice (would maybe reintroduce)
- Kombucha (would not reintroduce)
- Oolong tea (would not reintroduce)
- Soda pop (would not reintroduce)
- Soy milk (would not reintroduce)
- Sports drinks (would not reintroduce)
- Strong chai tea (would not reintroduce)
- Strong herbal tea
- Wine (would not reintroduce)

What you can eat on Paleo Low FODMAP Phase 1, 2, and 3:

Certain meat/protein

- Beef
- Chicken
- Eggs
- Lamb
- Pork
- Seafood
- Turkey

Certain vegetables

- Arugula
- Bell peppers
- Black olives
- Butternut squash
- Carrots
- Celery
- Cucumber
- Green olives
- Kale
- Lettuce
- Zucchini
- Oyster mushrooms
- Parsnip
- Spaghetti squash
- Spinach
- Summer squash
- Sweet potato (in small amounts)
- Swiss chard
- Tomatoes
- Turnips
- Water chestnuts

Certain fruit

- Banana
- Blueberries
- Lemons
- Limes
- Melons
- Oranges
- Papaya
- Passion fruit
- Pineapple
- Raspberries
- Strawberries

Certain seeds + nuts (always in moderation)

- Almonds (15 or less)
- Brazil nuts
- Chestnuts
- Chia seeds
- Hazelnuts (15 or less)
- Hemp seeds
- Macadamia nuts
- Peanuts
- Pecans (15 or less)
- Pine nuts (15 or less)
- Poppy seeds
- Pumpkin seeds
- Sunflower seeds
- Walnuts

Certain fats, oils, and vinegar

- Animal fat
- Apple cider vinegar
- Avocado oil
- Balsamic vinegar
- Macadamia nut oil
- Olive oil

Certain beverages
- Coffee (if you're allowing it on Paleo)
- Water
- Weak herbal tea (no apple)

RISKS WITH THE PALEO LOW FODMAP DIET

Every diet comes with downsides and risks; the Paleo LOw FODMAP diet is no exception. Some of the risks come from the Low Fodmap part, while others are more associated with going Paleo. Knowing the most common problems can help you avoid them and decide if this is the right eating lifestyle for you.

Risk #1: Changing too much too quickly

The first part of Paleo Low FODMAP is drastic, especially if you haven't been Paleo before. If you are Paleo, your body would have adjusted to eliminating grain, refined sugar, and other foods already, so you'll just be getting used to eliminating the high FODMAPs. However, even if you are starting out the Paleo Low FODMAP with a strong start, you can change too much too quickly. These changes aren't necessarily tied to food. Are you on new medications or other health protocols for your digestive disorder? Is it a busy time with family or work? Change, even good change, can be stressful, and stress can aggravate your GI symptoms. The benefits of the Paleo Low FODMAP diet may take longer, and this in itself is stressful. Pick a time in your life when things are relatively calm, and you can focus on taking it easy and taking care of yourself.

Risk #2: Micronutrient deficiencies

This is more of an issue with being Paleo, because on the basic Low FODMAP, most of the foods you eliminate come back after a set amount of time. When you're Paleo, however, you're eliminate entire food groups (like grain and dairy). All diets that eliminate so much are risky because of the nutrients you miss. Dairy is a source of calcium and Vitamin D. They are present in other foods, so you have to be intentional about getting them from places like dark leafy greens and fish. High-quality supplements might also be necessary, if a doctor/nutritionist finds your levels low.

Fiber is another nutrient many people don't get enough of when they're on the Paleo Low FODMAP diet. When the Low FODMAP diet starts, you eliminate a lot of sources of fiber in phase 1. This can be a real problem, since fiber is necessary for good gut health, and you're already dealing with a GI disorder. Normally, you add a lot of fiber sources back in during phase 2 and 3 of the Low FODMAP diet, but if you're Paleo, you don't. Low fiber intake is a very common downside of being Paleo, so be sure to get enough fibrous vegetables in place of grains, and check in with your doctor/nutritionist.

Risk #3: Disordered eating

The Low FODMAP diet starts out with a lot of rules and restrictions, but eventually loosens up. Being Paleo, however, requires a lot more attention. When you combine them, you have a recipe for disordered eating. What is that? It's an umbrella term for an obsession with food quality, anxiety around food, and more. Disordered eating can bloom into eating disorders like anorexia, but they aren't the same.

With the Paleo Low FODMAP, disordered eating can look like severe anxiety around food and worry about it causing symptoms; obsession with food labels and ingredients; and questioning if something is truly "Paleo." Essentially, food rules your life, even if you aren't counting calories or concerned with weight loss. You're fixated on the concept of "bad" and "good" food, and "clean" and "toxic" food. You might get more and more extreme with your diet, risking malnutrition, your social life, and peace of mind. All restrictive diets come with a risk of disordered eating, so be cautious.

How to succeed on the Paleo Low FODMAP diet

The Paleo Low FODMAP is kind of an odd duck of a diet, because the Low FODMAP part is short-term, while Paleo is long-term. It will be a very personalized diet based on what you learn during phase 2 about what high FODMAP foods to avoid. To develop the best diet and stick to it, there are certain steps you can take throughout all three phases:

Keep a symptom journal

During phase 1 and 2, how you feel directs your Paleo Low FODMAP diet. During the time you're eating Low FODMAPs and your body is resetting, your symptoms should gradually improve. Write down how you're feeling, your energy levels, and your mood. The more information you can collect, the better. During phase 2, when you start adding food back in, how you feel is also very important. Certain foods will aggravate your symptoms, and you'll want to record which ones and how much of the food you ate. This way, you know what to avoid or limit in the future. In this journal, you can also write down Paleo-friendly brands you find, so you aren't always trying to remember what's acceptable and always reading labels.

Meal plan

Planning meals saves a lot of time, energy, and even money for just about anybody, but it's especially useful for restrictive diets like Paleo. Meal-planning will be helpful during phase 1 and 2 of the Low FODMAP diet, since you're working with limited ingredients, and then specific ingredients as you add them back in. For phase 3, which will basically be a long-term Paleo that's modified to what foods don't aggravate your symptoms, keep up the meal-planning. You'll have complete control over what does or doesn't go into your meals, and with proper planning and prepping, you'll never be lost about what to make. Your fridge, pantry, and freezer will always be stocked. Most people like to meal plan about 4-5 days ahead or so, using ingredients from a weekly shopping trip, but if you have the time and freezer space, you can prep meals even further ahead than that.

In the long-term, think flexible

The Low FODMAP diet's most extreme aspects end in phase 3, but Paleo remains restrictive. To succeed long-term and be healthy, you have to be willing to be flexible. Being a strict Paleo may not end up being the healthiest choice, so you have to be willing to add certain foods back in (like grain and dairy) if it becomes necessary. Using your symptom journal, keep track of things like your energy level, skin health, GI symptoms, and so on. If you are concerned about something, talk to a professional and see what they recommend. Staying healthy is more important than sticking to a specific diet and its rules.

BREAKFAST RECIPES

Contents

Zucchini Sausage Casserole 22
Delicious Breakfast Bake 23
Turnip Dill Puree 24
Spinach Pepper Frittata 25
Italian Breakfast Sausage 26
Tasty Crab Cake Waffles 27
Mashed Potatoes 28
Salmon Waffles 29
Kale Pineapple Smoothie 30
Healthy Breakfast Frittata 31
Spinach Berry Smoothie 32
Kiwi Green Smoothie 33
Mint Pineapple Smoothie 34
Egg Scramble 35
Salmon Cakes 36
Choco Chia Pudding 37
Sauteed Shrimp 38
Breakfast Egg Muffins 39
Egg Bacon Muffins 40
Spinach Pepper Egg Bites 41
Zucchini Egg Muffins 42
Chicken Egg Muffins 43
Sausage Kale Egg Muffins 44
Pumpkin Smoothie 45
Spinach Basil Egg Scramble 46
Refreshing Kiwi Green Smoothie 47
Banana Strawberry Smoothie 48
Green Tropical Smoothie 49
Tuna Waffles 50
Delicious Pumpkin Scones 51

Zucchini Sausage Casserole

Serves: 8 / Preparation time: 10 minutes / Cooking time: 50 minutes

12 eggs

3 tomatoes, sliced

3 tbsp coconut flour

¼ cup coconut milk

2 small zucchinis, shredded

1 lb ground Italian sausage

¼ tsp pepper

½ tsp salt

- Preheat the oven to 350 F/ 180 C.
- Spray casserole dish with cooking spray and set aside.
- Cook Italian sausage in a pan until lightly brown. Transfer sausage to a large mixing bowl.
- Add coconut flour, milk, eggs, zucchini, pepper, and salt. Stir to mix.
- Add eggs and whisk until well combined.
- Transfer bowl mixture into the prepared casserole dish and top with tomato slices.
- Bake in preheated oven for 45-50 minutes.
- Serve and enjoy.

Per Serving: Calories: 319; Total Fat: 22.4g; Saturated Fat: 9g; Protein: 20.1g; Carbs: 7.8g; Fiber: 2.9g; Sugar: 3.9g

Delicious Breakfast Bake

Serves: 6 / Preparation time: 10 minutes / Cooking time: 45 minutes

10 eggs

2 large tomatoes, sliced

2 tbsp chives, chopped

3 cups baby spinach, chopped

1 tbsp ghee

10 bacon sliced, cooked and crumbled

½ tsp salt

- Preheat the oven to 350 F/ 180 C.
- Spray a 9-inch baking dish with cooking spray and set aside.
- Heat ghee in a medium pan. Add spinach and cook until spinach wilted.
- Whisk eggs and salt in mixing bowl. Add spinach and chives and whisk well.
- Pour egg mixture into the prepared baking dish.
- Top with bacon and tomatoes and bake for 40-45 minutes.
- Serve and enjoy.

Per Serving: Calories: 272; Total Fat: 21.3g; Saturated Fat: 7.8g; Protein: 18.6g; Carbs: 3.5g; Fiber: 1.1g; Sugar: 2.2g

Turnip Dill Puree

Serves: 4 / Preparation time: 10 minutes / Cooking time: 12 minutes

1 ½ lbs turnips, peeled and chopped

2 tbsp fresh chives, chopped

1 tsp dill

5 bacon slices, cooked and crumbled

- Add water and turnips in a large pot and cook for 12 minutes or until turnips is softened. Drain well and place in a food processor.
- Add dill and process until pureed, about 30 seconds.
- Transfer turnip puree in serving dish and top with chives and bacon.
- Serve and enjoy.

Per Serving: Calories: 178; Total Fat: 9.9g; Saturated Fat: 3.3g; Protein: 10.3g; Carbs: 11.7g; Fiber: 2.9g; Sugar: 7g

Spinach Pepper Frittata

Serves: 4 / Preparation time: 10 minutes / Cooking time: 15 minutes

10 eggs

1 cup spinach, chopped

1 bell pepper, diced

2 tbsp ghee

4 bacon slices

- Preheat the broiler.
- In a large bowl, whisk eggs until well combined and set aside.
- In a pan cook bacon. Once the bacon is cooked then diced and set aside.
- In same pan melt ghee. Add bell pepper and cook until softened.
- Add spinach and cook until spinach is wilted.
- Return bacon to the pan and stir well.
- Pour eggs over vegetable and bacon mixture and stir to mix.
- Cook frittata for 4 minutes then place the pan under the broiler and cook for 5 minutes more.
- Slice and serve.

Per Serving: Calories: 327; Total Fat: 25.4g; Saturated Fat: 10g; Protein: 21.4g; Carbs: 3.6g; Fiber: 0.6g; Sugar: 2.4g

Italian Breakfast Sausage

Serves: 6 / Preparation time: 10 minutes / Cooking time: 15 minutes

2 lbs ground pork

1 tsp fennel seed

1 tsp paprika

1 tsp red pepper flakes

1 tbsp dried parsley

1 ½ tbsp Italian seasoning

2 tbsp olive oil

2 tsp salt

- Preheat the oven to 375 F/ 190 C.
- Line baking tray with parchment paper and set aside.
- In a large bowl, combine together ground pork, fennel seed, paprika, red pepper flakes, parsley, Italian seasoning, olive oil, pepper, and salt.
- Make small even shape patties from meat mixture and place on a baking tray and bake in preheated oven for 15 minutes.
- Serve and enjoy.

Per Serving: Calories: 270; Total Fat: 11.2g; Saturated Fat: 2.7g; Protein: 39.7g; Carbs: 1g; Fiber: 0.4g; Sugar: 0.4g

Tasty Crab Cake Waffles

Serves: 4 / Preparation time: 10 minutes / Cooking time: 6 minutes

12 oz can wild-caught crab, drained

½ cup almond flour

1 tbsp paleo mayonnaise

1 tbsp lemon juice

1 tsp olive oil

2 tbsp fresh parsley, chopped

2 tbsp fresh chives, chopped

2 eggs, lightly beaten

- In a mixing bowl, mix together eggs, almond flour, mayo, lemon juice, oil, parsley, chives, and crab until well combined.
- Heat waffle maker according to the machine instructions.
- Divide waffle mixture into the four even patties.
- Place two patties on the hot waffle maker. Close and cook for 3 minutes. Repeat with remaining two.
- Serve and enjoy.

Per Serving: Calories: 230; Total Fat: 13.2g; Saturated Fat: 1.7g; Protein: 23.9g; Carbs: 5.1g; Fiber: 1.6g; Sugar: 1g

Mashed Potatoes

Serves: 6 / Preparation time: 10 minutes / Cooking time: 14 minutes

3 lbs potatoes, wash and cut into fourths

1 tbsp olive oil

4 tbsp chives, chopped

½ cup ghee

1 ¾ cups unsweetened coconut milk

1 ½ tsp salt

- Add 1 cup of water and potatoes in the instant pot.
- Cover pot with lid and cook on high pressure for 14 minutes.
- Once done release pressure using the quick release method then carefully remove the lid.
- Drain potatoes well and transfer in a large bowl.
- Add ghee, coconut milk, and salt and mash using potato masher until smooth.
- Add oil and chives and stir well.
- Serve and enjoy.

Per Serving: Calories: 488; Total Fat: 36.3g; Saturated Fat: 25.8g; Protein: 5.5g; Carbs: 39.6g; Fiber: 7g; Sugar: 5g

Salmon Waffles

Serves: 5 / Preparation time: 10 minutes / Cooking time: 9 minutes

12 oz can salmon, drained

½ cup almond flour

1 tbsp paleo mayonnaise

1 tbsp fresh lemon juice

1 tsp olive oil

2 tbsp green onion, chopped (green part only)

2 tbsp fresh dill, chopped

2 eggs, lightly beaten

½ tsp salt

- In a mixing bowl, mix together salmon, almond flour, mayo, lemon juice, oil, green onion, dill, eggs, and salt until well combined.
- Heat waffle maker according to the machine instructions.
- Make five even shape patties from the salmon mixture.
- Place two patties on the hot waffle maker. Cover and cook for 3 minutes. Repeat with remaining three.
- Serve and enjoy.

Per Serving: Calories: 208; Total Fat: 13.5g; Saturated Fat: 2.3g; Protein: 18.4g; Carbs: 4.2g; Fiber: 1.4g; Sugar: 0.9g

Kale Pineapple Smoothie

Serves: 1 / Preparation time: 5 minutes / Cooking time: 5 minutes

1 cup kale

¾ cup pineapple chunks

½ orange, skin removed

1 cup coconut milk

½ tsp ginger, grated

1 cup ice

- Add all ingredients into the blender and blend until smooth and creamy.
- Serve and enjoy.

Per Serving: Calories: 266; Total Fat: 12.3g; Saturated Fat: 10g; Protein: 5g; Carbs: 37.6g; Fiber: 5.1g; Sugar: 20.8g

Healthy Breakfast Frittata

Serves: 4 / Preparation time: 10 minutes / Cooking time: 15 minutes

6 eggs, lightly beaten

½ cup green onion, chopped (green part only)

1 bell pepper, chopped

2 tsp olive oil

1 tsp fresh oregano, chopped

Pepper

Salt

- Preheat the oven to 350 F/ 180 C.
- Whisk eggs in a bowl until well combined.
- Heat oil in a 10-inch pan over medium heat.
- Add bell pepper and sauté for 2 minutes. Add green onion and sauté for a minute. Season with pepper and salt.
- Pour egg mixture into the pan and cook over medium-low heat for 8 minutes.
- Place pan in the oven and bake for 5 minutes.
- Sprinkle oregano on top. Slice and serve.

Per Serving: Calories: 129; Total Fat: 9g; Saturated Fat: 2.4g; Protein: 8.9g; Carbs: 3.9g; Fiber: 0.9g; Sugar: 2.3g

Spinach Berry Smoothie

Serves: 1 / Preparation time: 5 minutes / Cooking time: 5 minutes

1 banana

2-inches cucumber, cubed

2 cups baby spinach

1 cup coconut milk

1 cup strawberries

- Add all ingredients into the blender and blend until smooth.
- Serve and enjoy.

Per Serving: Calories: 380; Total Fat: 13.7g; Saturated Fat: 10.4g; Protein: 9.3g; Carbs: 64.9g; Fiber: 10.3g; Sugar: 31.8g

Kiwi Green Smoothie

Serves: 2 / Preparation time: 5 minutes / Cooking time: 5 minutes

2 cups baby spinach

3/4 cucumber, diced

1 1/2 kiwi, peeled and chopped

2 cups ice cubes

- Add all ingredients into the blender and blend until smooth.
- Serve and enjoy.

Per Serving: Calories: 59; Total Fat: 0.5g; Saturated Fat: 0.1g; Protein: 2.2g; Carbs: 13.6g; Fiber: 2.9g; Sugar: 7.1g

Mint Pineapple Smoothie

Serves: 2 / Preparation time: 5 minutes / Cooking time: 5 minutes

3 cups fresh pineapple, cubed

1 ½ cups ice cubes

½ cup water

¼ cup fresh mint leaves

- Add all ingredients into the blender and blend until smooth.
- Serve and enjoy.

Per Serving: Calories: 128; Total Fat: 0.4g; Saturated Fat: 0g; Protein: 1.7g; Carbs: 33.4g; Fiber: 4.2g; Sugar: 24.4g

Egg Scramble

Serves: 2 / Preparation time: 5 minutes / Cooking time: 5 minutes

2 eggs, lightly beaten

2 tbsp fresh basil, chopped

1 tbsp olive oil

½ tomato, chopped

Pepper

Salt

- Heat oil in a pan over medium heat.
- Add tomatoes to the pan and cook until softened.
- Whisk eggs with basil, pepper, and salt.
- Add egg mixture to the pan and cook until eggs are done.
- Serve and enjoy.

Per Serving: Calories: 126; Total Fat: 11.4g; Saturated Fat: 2.4g; Protein: 5.8g; Carbs: 1g; Fiber: 0.2g; Sugar: 0.8g

Salmon Cakes

Serves: 5/ Preparation time: 10 minutes / Cooking time: 50 minutes

1 egg, lightly beaten

2 tbsp capers, drained

1 tbsp fresh lemon juice

2 tbsp dill, chopped

½ cup potato, boiled and mashed

12 oz salmon

¾ tsp salt

- Preheat the oven to 350 F/ 180 C.
- Place salmon on center of foil piece and season with salt. Wrap foil tightly around the salmon.
- Place salmon packet into the preheated oven and cook for 15-20 minutes.
- In a large bowl, shred the cooked salmon. Add mashed potatoes.
- Add remaining ingredients and mix until well combined.
- Make mini patties from salmon mixture and place onto the baking tray and bake for 25-30 minutes. Turn patties halfway through.
- Serve and enjoy.

Per Serving: Calories: 113; Total Fat: 5.2g; Saturated Fat: 0.9g; Protein: 14.8g; Carbs: 2.3g; Fiber: 0.5g; Sugar: 0.2g

Choco Chia Pudding

Serves: 4 / Preparation time: 5 minutes / Cooking time: 5 minutes

¼ cup chia seeds

1 ½ cups unsweetened coconut milk

½ tsp vanilla

½ tsp ground cinnamon

3 tbsp maple syrup

¼ cup unsweetened cocoa powder

Pinch of salt

- In a bowl, mix together cocoa powder, vanilla, cinnamon, maple syrup, and salt.
- Add coconut milk and whisk until smooth.
- Add chia seeds and whisk to combine. Cover and place in the refrigerator for 4-5 hours.
- Serve chilled and enjoy.

Per Serving: Calories: 295; Total Fat: 24.5g; Saturated Fat: 19.7g; Protein: 4.7g; Carbs: 19.8g; Fiber: 3.9g; Sugar: 12.1g

Sauteed Shrimp

Serves: 4 / Preparation time: 5 minutes / Cooking time: 5 minutes

1 lb shrimp

4 tbsp butter

1 lemon juice

½ tsp paprika

¼ tsp pepper

1 tsp Italian seasoning

½ tsp salt

- In a bowl, add shrimp, paprika, Italian seasoning, pepper, and salt. Toss well.
- Melt butter in a pan over medium heat.
- Add shrimp to the pan and cook for 2-3 minutes on each side.
- Drizzle lemon juice over shrimp and serve.

Per Serving: Calories: 241; Total Fat: 13.8g; Saturated Fat: 8g; Protein: 26g; Carbs: 2.1g; Fiber: 0.1g; Sugar: 0.1g

Breakfast Egg Muffins

Serves: 12 / Preparation time: 10 minutes / Cooking time: 20 minutes

12 eggs, lightly beaten

1 tsp Italian seasoning

1 cup fresh spinach, chopped

1 cup tomatoes, chopped

4 tbsp water

½ tsp pepper

¼ tsp salt

- Preheat the oven to 350 F/ 180 C.
- Spray a muffin tray with cooking spray and set aside.
- Whisk eggs in a medium bowl with water, Italian seasoning, pepper, and salt.
- Add spinach and tomatoes to the egg mixture and whisk well.
- Pour egg mixture into the prepared muffin tray and bake in preheated oven for 18-20 minutes.
- Serve and enjoy.

Per Serving: Calories: 68; Total Fat: 4.5g; Saturated Fat: 1.4g; Protein: 5.8g; Carbs: 1.1g; Fiber: 0.3g; Sugar: 0.8g

Egg Bacon Muffins

Serves: 12 / Preparation time: 10 minutes / Cooking time: 25 minutes

12 eggs, lightly beaten

2 green onion, chopped (green part only)

8 bacon slices, cooked and crumbled

2 tbsp fresh parsley, chopped

½ tsp dry mustard powder

1/3 cup unsweetened coconut milk

Pepper

Salt

- Preheat the oven to 375 F/ 190 C.
- Spray a muffin tray with cooking spray and set aside.
- In a bowl, whisk eggs with coconut milk, mustard, pepper, and salt until well combined.
- Add bacon, green onion, and parsley to the egg mixture and whisk well.
- Pour egg mixture into the muffin tray and bake in preheated oven for 20-25 minutes.
- Serve and enjoy.

Per Serving: Calories: 149; Total Fat: 11.3g; Saturated Fat: 4.5g; Protein: 10.5g; Carbs: 1.2g; Fiber: 0.3g; Sugar: 0.6g

Spinach Pepper Egg Bites

Serves: 12 / Preparation time: 10 minutes / Cooking time: 20 minutes

8 eggs

1 cup spinach, chopped

1 cup roasted red peppers, chopped

¼ cup unsweetened coconut milk

¼ cup green onion, chopped (green part only)

½ tsp salt

- Preheat the oven to 350 F/ 180 C.
- Spray a muffin tray with cooking spray and set aside.
- In a bowl, whisk eggs with coconut milk and salt.
- Add spinach, green onion, and red peppers to the egg mixture and stir to combine.
- Pour egg mixture into the prepared muffin tray and bake for 20 minutes.
- Serve and enjoy.

Per Serving: Calories: 59; Total Fat: 4.2g; Saturated Fat: 2g; Protein: 4.1g; Carbs: 1.7g; Fiber: 0.4g; Sugar: 1.1g

Zucchini Egg Muffins

Serves: 12 / Preparation time: 10 minutes / Cooking time: 20 minutes

8 eggs

12 bacon slices, cooked and crumbled

2 small zucchini, sliced

¼ cup coconut milk

2 tbsp parsley, chopped

1 cup baby spinach, chopped

1 red bell pepper, diced

¼ cup green onion, chopped (green part only)

1 tbsp olive oil

Pepper

Salt

- Preheat the oven to 350 F/ 180 C.
- Spray a muffin tray with cooking spray and set aside.
- Heat olive oil in a pan over medium heat. Add parsley, spinach, green onion, red bell pepper to the pan and sauté until spinach is wilted.
- In a bowl, whisk eggs with coconut milk, pepper, and salt.
- Add sautéed vegetables, bacon, and zucchini to the egg mixture and stir well.
- Pour egg mixture into the prepared muffin tray and bake in preheated oven for 20 minutes.
- Serve and enjoy.

Per Serving: Calories: 164; Total Fat: 12.1g; Saturated Fat: 4.6g; Protein: 11.3g; Carbs: 2.5g; Fiber: 0.6g; Sugar: 1.3g

Chicken Egg Muffins

Serves: 12 / Preparation time: 10 minutes / Cooking time: 15 minutes

10 eggs

1 cup chicken, cooked and chopped

1/3 cup green onions, chopped (green part only)

¼ tsp pepper

1 tsp sea salt

- Preheat the oven to 400 F/ 200 C.
- Spray a muffin tray with cooking spray and set aside.
- In a large bowl, whisk eggs with pepper and salt.
- Add remaining ingredients and stir well.
- Pour egg mixture into the prepared muffin tray and bake in preheated oven for 14-15 minutes.
- Serve and enjoy.

Per Serving: Calories: 71; Total Fat: 4g; Saturated Fat: 1.2g; Protein: 8g; Carbs: 0.5g; Fiber: 0.1g; Sugar: 0.3g

Sausage Kale Egg Muffins

Serves: 12 / Preparation time: 10 minutes / Cooking time: 35 minutes

10 eggs

¼ cup kale, chopped

¼ cup sun-dried tomatoes, chopped

1 cup coconut milk

¼ cup sausage, sliced

Pepper

Salt

- Preheat the oven to 350 F/ 180 C.
- Spray a muffin tray with cooking spray and set aside.
- In a large bowl, add all ingredients and whisk until well combined.
- Pour egg mixture into the prepared muffin tray and bake for 30-35 minutes or until eggs are set.
- Serve and enjoy.

Per Serving: Calories: 115; Total Fat: 9.8g; Saturated Fat: 5.8g; Protein: 5.7g; Carbs: 2g; Fiber: 0.5g; Sugar: 1.2g

Pumpkin Smoothie

Serves: 2 / Preparation time: 5 minutes / Cooking time: 5 minutes

½ tsp pumpkin pie spice

1 tbsp maple syrup

1 cup unsweetened coconut milk

1/3 cup pumpkin puree

1 frozen banana

1 scoop vanilla protein powder

- Add all ingredients into the blender and blend until smooth.
- Serve and enjoy.

Per Serving: Calories: 425; Total Fat: 29g; Saturated Fat: 25.6g; Protein: 17.4g; Carbs: 30.7g; Fiber: 5.7g; Sugar: 18.7g

Spinach Basil Egg Scramble

Serves: 2 / Preparation time: 10 minutes / Cooking time: 10 minutes

4 eggs

1 ½ cups baby spinach, chopped

1/3 cup basil, chopped

1 tbsp olive oil

3 tomatoes, chopped

Pepper

Salt

- Heat oil in a pan over medium heat.
- Add tomatoes and cook until softened.
- Meanwhile, in a bowl, whisk eggs with basil, pepper, and salt.
- Add spinach to the pan and cook until wilted.
- Pour egg mixture to the pan and cook until eggs are done.
- Serve and enjoy.

Per Serving: Calories: 225; Total Fat: 16.2g; Saturated Fat: 3.8g; Protein: 13.5g; Carbs: 8.8g; Fiber: 2.8g; Sugar: 5.6g

Refreshing Kiwi Green Smoothie

Serves: 2 / Preparation time: 5 minutes / Cooking time: 5 minutes

2 cups fresh spinach

4 kiwis, peeled

1 banana, peeled

7 oz cucumber, diced

- Add all ingredients into the blender and blend until smooth.
- Serve and enjoy.

Per Serving: Calories: 167; Total Fat: 1.2g; Saturated Fat: 0.2g; Protein: 3.9g; Carbs: 40.5g; Fiber: 7.3g; Sugar: 22.7g

Banana Strawberry Smoothie

Serves: 1 / Preparation time: 5 minutes / Cooking time: 5 minutes

½ banana

1 tsp maple syrup

¾ cup unsweetened coconut milk

5 strawberries

- Add all ingredients into the blender and blend until smooth.
- Serve and enjoy.

Per Serving: Calories: 134; Total Fat: 4.4g; Saturated Fat: 4.1g; Protein: 1g; Carbs: 24.6g; Fiber: 3.7g; Sugar: 14.1g

Green Tropical Smoothie

Serves: 1 / Preparation time: 5 minutes / Cooking time: 5 minutes

1 cup coconut milk

½ tsp ground ginger

½ tbsp lime juice

1 cup baby spinach

¾ cup pineapple chunks

1 tbsp flaxseed

Pinch of salt

- Add all ingredients into the blender and blend until smooth and creamy.
- Serve and enjoy.

Per Serving: Calories: 234; Total Fat: 14.5g; Saturated Fat: 10.3g; Protein: 4.3g; Carbs: 22.8g; Fiber: 4.4g; Sugar: 12.5g

Tuna Waffles

Serves: 4 / Preparation time: 10 minutes / Cooking time: 8 minutes

10 oz can tuna, drained

½ cup sunflower seed flour

1 tbsp chives, chopped

2 eggs, lightly beaten

1 tbsp olive oil

1 tbsp fresh lemon juice

1 tbsp paleo mayonnaise

¼ tsp salt

- In a bowl, combine together tuna, sunflower seed flour, chives, eggs, oil, lemon juice, mayonnaise, and salt.
- Heat waffle maker according to the machine instructions.
- Make four even shape patties from the mixture.
- Place two patties onto the hot waffle maker. Cover and cook for 4 minutes. Repeat with remaining two.
- Serve and enjoy.

Per Serving: Calories: 185; Total Fat: 7.7g; Saturated Fat: 1.6g; Protein: 24.8g; Carbs: 4g; Fiber: 0.5g; Sugar: 0.5g

Delicious Pumpkin Scones

Serves: 8 / Preparation time: 10 minutes / Cooking time: 22 minutes

¾ tsp pumpkin pie spice

½ tsp cinnamon

1 tsp vanilla

2 tbsp almond milk

2 tbsp maple syrup

¼ cup coconut sugar

1 egg

½ cup pumpkin puree

6 tbsp butter, cubed

½ tsp baking soda

2 tsp baking powder

½ cup almond flour

¾ cup cassava flour

½ tsp salt

- Preheat the oven to 350 F/ 180 C.
- Line baking tray with parchment paper and set aside.
- In a mixing bowl, mix together almond flour, cassava flour, baking soda, baking powder, salt, and butter.
- Whisk together egg, pumpkin pie spice, vanilla, coconut milk, maple syrup, coconut sugar, and pumpkin puree.
- Pour dry ingredients mixture into the wet ingredients mixture and mix well with hand. Let sit dough for 5 minutes.
- Mold the dough into a 6-inch circle and cut into eight triangles. Transfer scones on a prepared baking tray and bake for 22 minutes.
- Serve and enjoy.

Per Serving: Calories: 189; Total Fat: 13.7g; Saturated Fat: 6.7g; Protein: 2.6g; Carbs: 15.9g; Fiber: 1.5g; Sugar: 10g

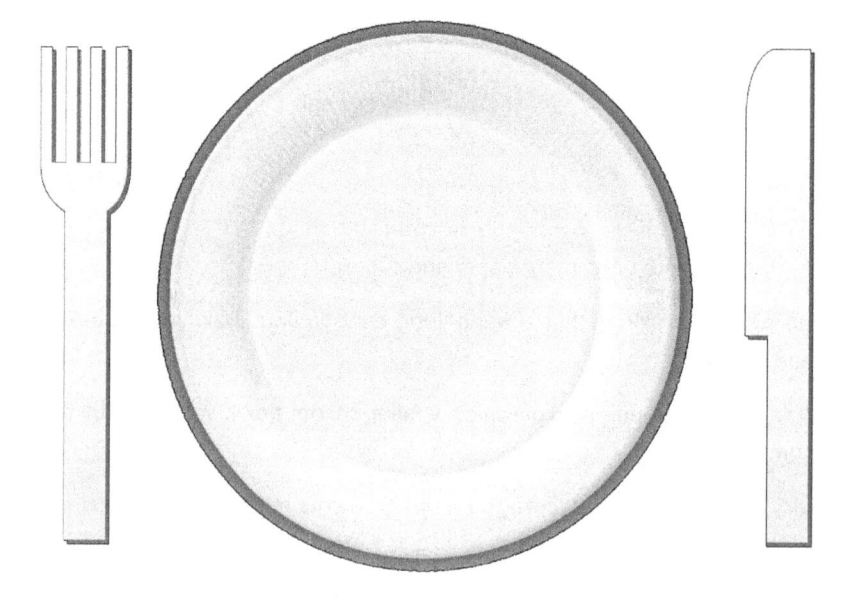

LUNCH RECIPES

Contents

Flavorful Chicken Salad 54
Greek Chicken Salad 55
Chicken Berry Salad 56
Potato Salad 57
Tomato Chicken Soup 58
Pulled Pork 59
Turkey Meatballs 60
Flavors Picadillo 61
Zucchini Chicken Meatballs 62
Delicious Pepper Soup 63
Easy Pesto Chicken Salad 64
Meat Patties 65
Chicken Chili 66
Chicken Chili Soup 67
Chicken Zoodle Soup 68
Cucumber Tomato Salad 69
Curried Chicken Soup 70
Coconut Fish Stew 71
Summer Veggie Soup 72
Delicious Chicken Green Chile 73
Healthy Kale Salad 74
Strawberry kale Salad 75
Herb Zucchini Noodles 76
Lemon Chicken Salad 77
Green Beans with Pine Nuts 78
Easy Egg Salad 79
Roasted Veggies 80
Easy Braised Turnips 81
Italian Meatball Soup 82
Classic Antipasto Salad 83

Flavorful Chicken Salad

Serves: 4 / Preparation time: 10 minutes / Cooking time: 10 minutes

1 ½ cups chicken, cooked and diced

1 tsp Dijon mustard

2 tsp olive oil

1 tsp vinegar

½ cup paleo mayonnaise

¼ cup almonds, sliced

1/3 cup green onion, sliced (green parts only)

1/3 cup bell pepper, diced

1 cup fresh pineapple, diced

Pepper

Salt

- Add chicken, green onion, almonds, bell pepper, and pineapple in a large mixing bowl and stir to combine.
- For the dressing: In a small bowl, whisk together mayonnaise, mustard, oil, vinegar, pepper, and salt.
- Pour dressing over chicken mixture and stir to combine.
- Serve and enjoy.

Per Serving: Calories: 276; Total Fat: 16.8g; Saturated Fat: 2.5g; Protein: 17.3g; Carbs: 15.2g; Fiber: 1.7g; Sugar: 6.9g

Greek Chicken Salad

Serves: 4 / Preparation time: 10 minutes / Cooking time: 15 minutes

1 ½ lbs chicken breast

¼ cup dried oregano

2 tbsp vinegar

½ cup fresh lemon juice

½ cup olive oil

½ tsp pepper

2 tsp salt

For Salad:

¼ cup green onion, chopped (green part only)

1 bell pepper, chopped

1 cucumber, chopped

½ cup olives, halved

2 cups cherry tomatoes, halved

3 romaine hearts, chopped

- In a bowl, whisk together olive oil, oregano, vinegar, lemon juice, pepper, and salt.
- Place chicken in a large bowl and pour half olive oil mixture over chicken. Cover and place in the refrigerator for overnight.
- Place the romaine in a large mixing bowl and top with all the vegetables.
- Heat pan over medium heat. Add marinated chicken to the pan and cook for 3-4 minutes on each side or until chicken is completely cooked.
- Cut chicken into the slices and place on the salad.
- Pour remaining olive oil mixture over salad and serve.

Per Serving: Calories: 492; Total Fat: 32.3g; Saturated Fat: 4.3g; Protein: 38.7g; Carbs: 13.8g; Fiber: 4.7g; Sugar: 6.1g

Chicken Berry Salad

Serves: 6 / Preparation time: 10 minutes / Cooking time: 5 minutes

2 lbs chicken, cooked and cut into bite-size pieces

3 tbsp chives, chopped

1 cup paleo mayonnaise

1 cup blueberries

1 lb strawberries, chopped

¼ tsp salt

- In a large mixing bowl, mix together chicken, chives, blueberries, strawberries, mayonnaise, and salt until well coated.
- Cover and place in the refrigerator for 1-2 hours.
- Serve chilled and enjoy.

Per Serving: Calories: 420; Total Fat: 18g; Saturated Fat: 3.2g; Protein: 44.9g; Carbs: 18.7g; Fiber: 2.1g; Sugar: 8.6g

Potato Salad

Serves: 4 / Preparation time: 10 minutes / Cooking time: 15 minutes

1 ½ lbs potatoes, diced

1 tsp vinegar

¼ tsp dried dill

½ tsp celery salt

1 tbsp yellow mustard

5 tbsp paleo mayonnaise

½ cup of water

- Add water and potatoes into the instant pot.
- Cover with lid and select steam mode and cook on high mode for 10 minutes.
- Meanwhile, in a large bowl, mix together remaining ingredients.
- Release instant pot pressure using the quick-release method then carefully remove the lid.
- Drain potatoes well and place into the large bowl.
- Stir well and serve.

Per Serving: Calories: 234; Total Fat: 12.8g; Saturated Fat: 1.9g; Protein: 3.1g; Carbs: 27.1g; Fiber: 4.3g; Sugar: 2.1g

Tomato Chicken Soup

Serves: 6 / Preparation time: 10 minutes / Cooking time: 28 minutes

30 oz can roasted tomatoes	1/3 cup fresh basil
14 oz coconut milk	1 cup water
2 lbs chicken thighs, skinless and boneless	¼ tsp pepper
2 tbsp olive oil	1 tsp salt

- Add tomatoes, chicken, olive oil, basil, water, pepper, and salt in the instant pot and stir well.
- Seal pot with a lid and select manual and set timer for 23 minutes.
- Once done then release pressure using quick-release method than open the lid.
- Remove chicken from pot and cut into small chunks.
- Using immersion blender blends the soup.
- Add chicken and coconut milk into the pot and stir well and cook on sauté mode for 5 minutes.
- Serve and enjoy.

Per Serving: Calories: 515; Total Fat: 31.7g; Saturated Fat: 17.7g; Protein: 46.5g; Carbs: 10.7g; Fiber: 3.8g; Sugar: 5.7g

Pulled Pork

Serves: 6 / Preparation time: 10 minutes / Cooking time: 50 minutes

3 lbs pork butt, cut into large chunks

6 tbsp water

½ tsp cayenne pepper

1 tbsp oregano

½ tsp cumin

2 tbsp smoked paprika

1 tbsp olive oil

1 tsp pepper

2 tsp salt

- Add meat into the instant pot and top with olive oil.
- In a small bowl, mix together paprika, cayenne, oregano, cumin, pepper, and salt and sprinkle over meat. Add water and stir well.
- Seal pot with a lid and select manual mode and set timer for 40 minutes.
- Once done then allow to release pressure naturally for 10 minutes then release using quick-release method.
- Remove meat from pot and shred using a fork.
- Return shredded meat to the pot and cook on sauté mode for 10 minutes more.
- Serve and enjoy.

Per Serving: Calories: 469; Total Fat: 17.9g; Saturated Fat: 5.4g; Protein: 71.1g; Carbs: 2.2g; Fiber: 1.3g; Sugar: 0.3g

Turkey Meatballs

Serves: 6 / Preparation time: 10 minutes / Cooking time: 25 minutes

1 lb ground turkey

2 tbsp chives, chopped

2 tbsp coconut flour

1 tsp olive oil

½ tsp ground ginger

1 egg, lightly beaten

½ tsp salt

- Preheat the oven to 375 F/ 190 C.
- In a large bowl, combine together turkey, chives, coconut flour, olive oil, ginger, egg, and salt until well combined.
- Make small even shape balls from meat mixture and place onto the baking tray.
- Bake meatballs in preheated oven for 23-25 minutes.
- Serve and enjoy.

Per Serving: Calories: 185; Total Fat: 10.5g; Saturated Fat: 2.4g; Protein: 22.3g; Carbs: 2.9g; Fiber: 1.7g; Sugar: 0.4g

Flavors Picadillo

Serves: 6 / Preparation time: 10 minutes / Cooking time: 20 minutes

2 lbs ground beef

½ cup green olives

1 tsp ground cumin

½ cup green onion, chopped (green part only)

14 oz can roasted tomatoes, blended

2 cups cherry tomatoes, halved

1 bell pepper, diced

1 tbsp olive oil

1 tsp salt

- In a large pan, brown the meat in the olive oil over medium heat. Season with salt and cook for 5 minutes.
- Add cumin, green onion, tomatoes, and bell pepper and cook for 10 minutes.
- Add olives and cook for 3-5 minutes more.
- Serve and enjoy.

Per Serving: Calories: 351; Total Fat: 13.2g; Saturated Fat: 4.1g; Protein: 47.4g; Carbs: 8.5g; Fiber: 2.7g; Sugar: 4.4g

Zucchini Chicken Meatballs

Serves: 6 / Preparation time: 10 minutes / Cooking time: 18 minutes

1 ½ cups zucchini, grated

1 ½ tsp Italian seasoning

2 tbsp chives, chopped

¼ cup almond flour

1 egg, lightly beaten

1 lb ground chicken

½ tsp salt

- Preheat the oven to 350 F/ 180 C.
- Line baking tray with parchment paper and set aside.
- Squeeze out all liquid from grated zucchini and place in a large bowl.
- Add chicken, seasoning, chives, egg, almond flour, and salt and mix until well combined.
- Make small even shape balls from meat mixture and place onto a baking tray.
- Bake in preheated oven for 18 minutes.
- Serve and enjoy.

Per Serving: Calories: 189; Total Fat: 9.1g; Saturated Fat: 2g; Protein: 24.2g; Carbs: 2.2g; Fiber: 0.8g; Sugar: 0.8g

Delicious Pepper Soup

Serves: 8 / Preparation time: 10 minutes / Cooking time: 20 minutes

- 2 lbs ground beef
- 3 cups cooked rice
- ½ cup water
- ½ cup green onion, chopped (green part only)
- 3 bell peppers, chopped
- 1 cup tomatoes, chopped
- 28 oz can roasted tomatoes, diced
- 2 tsp Italian seasoning
- 2 tbsp olive oil
- 1 tsp salt

- Heat oil in a large saucepan over medium heat.
- Add pepper and cook for 5 minutes or until tender.
- Add meat seasoning, and salt and cook until browned, about 5-7 minutes.
- Add tomatoes, water, and green onion and cook for 10 minutes.
- Add cooked rice and stir well.
- Serve hot and enjoy.

Per Serving: Calories: 542; Total Fat: 11.6g; Saturated Fat: 3.4g; Protein: 40.9g; Carbs: 65.2g; Fiber: 3.5g; Sugar: 5.6g

Easy Pesto Chicken Salad

Serves: 4 / Preparation time: 10 minutes / Cooking time: 5 minutes

1 ½ lbs chicken, cooked and cut into small chunks

½ cup paleo pesto

2/3 cup paleo mayonnaise

¼ cup cherry tomatoes, halved

- Add chicken to a large mixing bowl and add pesto and mayo. Stir well.
- Add cherry tomatoes and stir.
- Serve and enjoy.

Per Serving: Calories: 547; Total Fat: 31.3g; Saturated Fat: 5.9g; Protein: 52.7g; Carbs: 11.8g; Fiber: 0.6g; Sugar: 4.8g

Meat Patties

Serves: 6 / Preparation time: 10 minutes / Cooking time: 10 minutes

- 1 lb ground lamb
- 1 lb ground beef
- ½ cup green onion, chopped (green part only)
- 2 tbsp olive oil
- 1 tsp dried rosemary
- 1 tbsp dried oregano
- 1 tbsp dried thyme
- 1 tsp cumin
- 1 tsp pepper
- 1 ½ tsp salt

- Add all ingredients into the large bowl and mix until well combined.
- Make six even shape patties from meat mixture.
- Grill patties over medium heat for 5 minutes on each side.
- Serve and enjoy.

Per Serving: Calories: 330; Total Fat: 15.2g; Saturated Fat: 4.5g; Protein: 44.5g; Carbs: 1.9g; Fiber: 0.9g; Sugar: 0.2g

Chicken Chili

Serves: 6 / Preparation time: 10 minutes / Cooking time: 12 minutes

1 lb chicken thighs, skinless and boneless

½ tsp cumin

1 tsp chili powder

¼ tsp pepper

4 cups water

2 medium potatoes, chopped

2 tbsp olive oil

1 tsp salt

- Add all ingredients into the instant pot and stir well.
- Seal pot with lid and cook on manual high pressure for 12 minutes.
- Release pressure using the quick release method than open the lid.
- Remove chicken from pot and shred using a fork.
- Using immersion blender blends the soup until just chunky.
- Return shredded chicken to the pot and stir well.
- Serve and enjoy.

Per Serving: Calories: 235; Total Fat: 10.5g; Saturated Fat: 2.2g; Protein: 23.2g; Carbs: 11.5g; Fiber: 1.9g; Sugar: 0.9g

Chicken Chili Soup

Serves: 6 / Preparation time: 10 minutes / Cooking time: 5 minutes

2 lbs chicken breast, skinless, boneless, and cut in half

1 tbsp paprika

2 tsp cumin

1 tbsp oregano

2 tbsp olive oil

¼ cup green onion, chopped (green part only)

4 oz can green chilies, chopped

1 cup water

24 oz can tomatoes, diced

- Place chicken in the instant pot.
- Add tomatoes, paprika, cumin, oregano, olive oil, green onion, green chilies, water, pepper, and salt and stir well.
- Seal pot with lid and cook on manual mode for 10 minutes.
- Once done then allow to release pressure naturally for 10 minutes then release using quick-release method.
- Remove chicken from pot and cut into small chunks.
- Return chicken to the pot and stir well.
- Serve and enjoy.

Per Serving: Calories: 250; Total Fat: 8.9g; Saturated Fat: 0.7g; Protein: 33.7g; Carbs: 8.4g; Fiber: 3.2g; Sugar: 4.1g

Chicken Zoodle Soup

Serves: 8 / Preparation time: 10 minutes / Cooking time: 13 minutes

3 lbs chicken thighs, skinless and boneless

¼ cup green onion, chopped (green part only)

4 zucchini, spiralized using a slicer

1 cup unsweetened coconut milk

2 cups cherry tomatoes, halved

½ cup paleo pesto

2 cups water

1 tsp salt

- Add chicken, water, and salt into the instant pot and stir well.
- Cover pot with lid and cook on manual high pressure for 8 minutes.
- Once done then release pressure using the quick release method then carefully open the lid.
- Remove chicken from pot and cut into small chunks.
- Add green onion, zucchini, coconut milk, tomatoes, and pesto to the pot and stir well and cook on sauté mode for 5 minutes.
- Return chicken to the pot and stir well.
- Serve and enjoy.

Per Serving: Calories: 484; Total Fat: 26.5g; Saturated Fat: 11.1g; Protein: 53.1g; Carbs: 7.9g; Fiber: 2.6g; Sugar: 5g

Cucumber Tomato Salad

Serves: 5 / Preparation time: 10 minutes / Cooking time: 5 minutes

3 cups cherry tomatoes, halved

3 cups cucumbers, diced

2 tsp Italian seasoning

1 tbsp apple cider vinegar

2 tbsp olive oil

¼ cup green onion, chopped (green part only)

½ tsp salt

- Add all ingredients into the large mixing bowl and toss well.
- Cover and place in the refrigerator for 1-2 hours.
- Serve and enjoy.

Per Serving: Calories: 85; Total Fat: 6.5g; Saturated Fat: 0.9g; Protein: 1.5g; Carbs: 7.1g; Fiber: 1.7g; Sugar: 4.2g

Curried Chicken Soup

Serves: 6 / Preparation time: 10 minutes / Cooking time: 15 minutes

2 lbs chicken thighs

14 oz coconut milk

1 tsp ginger powder

3 tbsp curry powder

2 tbsp olive oil

2 cups water

¼ cup green onion, chopped (green part only)

14 oz can roasted tomatoes, diced

1 ½ lbs potatoes, chopped

12 oz carrots, chopped

1 ½ tsp salt

- Add chicken, ginger, curry powder, oil, water, green onion, tomatoes, potatoes, carrots, pepper, and salt into the instant pot and stir well.
- Seal pot with lid and cook on manual mode for 10 minutes.
- Once done then allow to release pressure naturally for 10 minutes then release using quick-release method than open the lid.
- Remove chicken from pot and cut into small chunks.
- Add coconut milk in soup mixture and stir well.
- Using an immersion blender blend the soup.
- Return chicken to the pot and stir well and cook soup on sauté mode for 5 minutes more.
- Serve and enjoy.

Per Serving: Calories: 610; Total Fat: 32.2g; Saturated Fat: 17.8g; Protein: 48.7g; Carbs: 32.6g; Fiber: 7.9g; Sugar: 8.1g

Coconut Fish Stew

Serves: 6 / Preparation time: 10 minutes / Cooking time: 15 minutes

2 lbs white fish fillets

¼ tsp red pepper flakes

2 cups water

14 oz coconut milk

14 oz can roasted tomatoes, diced

¼ cup green onion, chopped (green part only)

2 red bell peppers, chopped

2 tbsp olive oil

1 tsp salt

- Heat oil in a large pan over medium heat.
- Add green onion and bell peppers and cook for 5 minutes.
- Add fish, water, milk, and tomatoes and cook for 10 minutes or until fish is cooked.
- Add red pepper flakes and serve.

Per Serving: Calories: 483; Total Fat: 31.9g; Saturated Fat: 16.4g; Protein: 39.5g; Carbs: 10.3g; Fiber: 3.2g; Sugar: 5.9g

Summer Veggie Soup

Serves: 6 / Preparation time: 10 minutes / Cooking time: 40 minutes

3 large zucchini, chopped

6 cups water

½ cup green onion, chopped (green part only)

2 cups bell pepper, chopped

1 lb carrots, diced

3 large tomatoes, chopped

2 lbs ground Italian sausage

1 tsp salt

- Add sausage in a large saucepan and cook over medium heat until browned.
- Add tomatoes, water, green onion, bell peppers, carrots, and salt and bring to boil over medium-high heat.
- Turn heat to medium-low. Cover and cook for 20 minutes.
- Add zucchini and cook for 10 minutes more.
- Serve and enjoy.

Per Serving: Calories: 542; Total Fat: 35.3g; Saturated Fat: 12.1g; Protein: 30.6g; Carbs: 22.7g; Fiber: 5.5g; Sugar: 13.8g

Delicious Chicken Green Chile

Serves: 5 / Preparation time: 10 minutes / Cooking time: 6 hours

- 1 lb chicken breasts, skinless and boneless
- ½ tsp paprika
- ½ tsp dried sage
- ½ tsp cumin
- 1 tsp dried oregano
- 14 oz can tomatoes, diced
- 2 cups water
- 1 jalapeno pepper, chopped
- 1 poblano pepper, chopped
- 12 oz can green chilies
- ½ cup dried chives
- 1 tsp sea salt

- Add all ingredients into the slow cooker and stir well.
- Cover and cook on low for 6 hours.
- Remove chicken from slow cooker and shred using a fork.
- Return chicken to the slow cooker and stir well.
- Serve and enjoy.

Per Serving: Calories: 211; Total Fat: 7.1g; Saturated Fat: 1.9g; Protein: 27.9g; Carbs: 8.7g; Fiber: 3g; Sugar: 3.4g

Healthy Kale Salad

Serves: 8 / Preparation time: 10 minutes / Cooking time: 5 minutes

10 oz kale, rinsed and chopped

½ tsp cumin

½ jalapeno pepper, chopped

1 tbsp olive oil

4 tbsp fresh lime juice

¼ tsp sea salt

- Add kale into a large mixing bowl.
- In a small bowl, whisk together lime juice, cumin, jalapeno, oil, and salt and pour over kale.
- Toss well and serve.

Per Serving: Calories: 34; Total Fat: 1.8g; Saturated Fat: 0.3g; Protein: 1.1g; Carbs: 3.9g; Fiber: 0.6g; Sugar: 0g

Strawberry kale Salad

Serves: 4 / Preparation time: 10 minutes / Cooking time: 5 minutes

5 cups kale, chopped

3 tbsp pecans, chopped

1 ½ cups strawberries, sliced

For dressing:

½ tsp Dijon mustard

1 tsp maple syrup

1 tsp lemon zest

1 fresh lemon juice

1/3 cup olive oil

- Add kale, pecans, and strawberries in a large bowl.
- In a small bowl, whisk together all dressing ingredients and pour over salad.
- Toss well and serve.

Per Serving: Calories: 210; Total Fat: 17.1g; Saturated Fat: 2.5g; Protein: 3g; Carbs: 14.4g; Fiber: 2.4g; Sugar: 3.9g

Herb Zucchini Noodles

Serves: 4 / Preparation time: 10 minutes / Cooking time: 15 minutes

2 lbs zucchini, spiralized using a slicer

1 lb green beans, trimmed and cut into 1-inch pieces

½ cup olive oil

½ fresh lemon juice

½ cup basil leaves

1 tbsp thyme

4 tbsp chives, sliced

½ cup parsley

¼ cup sunflower seeds, toasted

Pepper

Salt

- Add herbs into the food processor and process until chopped.
- Add 6 tbsp oil and lemon juice and process until smooth. Season with pepper and salt.
- Add water in a large pot and bring to boil. Add green beans to the pot and cook for 5 minutes. Drain well and pat dry with paper towels.
- Heat remaining oil in a pan over medium heat.
- Add sunflower seeds and sauté for a minute. Remove seeds from the pan and set aside.
- Add herb mixture and green beans in a pan and sauté for 2-3 minutes.
- Add zucchini and sunflower seeds and cook for 1-2 minutes.
- Garnish with chives and serve.

Per Serving: Calories: 311; Total Fat: 27.4g; Saturated Fat: 3.9g; Protein: 5.9g; Carbs: 17.4g; Fiber: 7.2g; Sugar: 5.7g

Lemon Chicken Salad

Serves: 6 / Preparation time: 10 minutes / Cooking time: 5 minutes

2 lbs chicken, cooked and chopped

½ cup pineapple, chopped

2 tbsp chives, chopped

3 tbsp fresh lemon juice

1 lemon zest

½ tbsp poppy seeds

1 tbsp olive oil

½ cup paleo mayonnaise

¼ tsp pepper

½ tsp salt

- Add all ingredients into the large mixing bowl and stir everything well.
- Serve and enjoy.

Per Serving: Calories: 338; Total Fat: 13.9g; Saturated Fat: 2.7g; Protein: 44.3g; Carbs: 6.9g; Fiber: 0.3g; Sugar: 2.9g

Green Beans with Pine Nuts

Serves: 4 / Preparation time: 10 minutes / Cooking time: 5 minute

1 ¼ lbs green beans, washed and trimmed

½ lemon juice

1 tsp lemon zest

2 tbsp olive oil

¼ cup pine nuts

Pepper

Salt

- Add pine nuts in a pan and cook over medium-low heat for 3-4 minutes. Remove from heat and set aside.
- Add water in a large pot and bring to boil.
- In a small bowl, whisk together oil, lemon juice, lemon zest, pepper, and salt and set aside.
- Once the pot of water starts boiling then add green beans and cook for 2-3 minutes. Drain green beans and transfer to a large bowl.
- Pour dressing over green beans and toss well.
- Sprinkle pine nuts on top and serve.

Per Serving: Calories: 163; Total Fat: 13g; Saturated Fat: 1.5g; Protein: 3.8g; Carbs: 11.5g; Fiber: 5.2g; Sugar: 2.4g

Easy Egg Salad

Serves: 2 / Preparation time: 10 minutes / Cooking time: 5 minutes

4 hard-boiled eggs, chopped

1/8 tsp paprika

1 tbsp chives, minced

2 ½ tbsp bell pepper, minced

½ tsp Dijon mustard

3 tbsp paleo mayonnaise

Pepper

Salt

- Add all ingredients into the mixing bowl and stir well to mix.
- Serve and enjoy.

Per Serving: Calories: 261; Total Fat: 16.6g; Saturated Fat: 3.8g; Protein: 12.9g; Carbs: 17.4g; Fiber: 2.1g; Sugar: 9.6g

Roasted Veggies

Serves: 4 / Preparation time: 10 minutes / Cooking time: 1 hour 30 minutes

2 medium potatoes, cut into small pieces

1 small rutabaga, peeled and cut into small pieces

2 medium parsnips, peeled and cut into small pieces

3 medium carrots, peeled and cut into small pieces

¼ cup olive oil

Pepper

Salt

- Preheat the oven to 350 F/ 180 C.
- In a large bowl, toss vegetable with olive oil.
- Transfer vegetables on a baking tray and season with pepper and salt.
- Bake in preheated oven for 45 minutes.
- Stir well and bake for 45 minutes more.
- Serve and enjoy.

Per Serving: Calories: 246; Total Fat: 12.9g; Saturated Fat: 1.9g; Protein: 3.3g; Carbs: 32g; Fiber: 6.5g; Sugar: 8.1g

Easy Braised Turnips

Serves: 4 / Preparation time: 10 minutes / Cooking time: 10 minute

1 lb baby turnips, peeled and quartered

¾ cup low-FODMAP vegetable broth

2 tsp fresh thyme, chopped

3 tbsp ghee

2 tbsp green onion, chopped (green part only)

Pepper

Salt

- Melt ghee in large pan over medium heat.
- Add turnips, broth, thyme, pepper, and salt. Stir well.
- Cover and cook until turnips are tender, about 4 minutes.
- Remove cover and turn heat to high and cook for 5 minutes more.
- Serve and enjoy.

Per Serving: Calories: 126; Total Fat: 9.9g; Saturated Fat: 6g; Protein: 2g; Carbs: 8.2g; Fiber: 2.1g; Sugar: 257g

Italian Meatball Soup

Serves: 6 / Preparation time: 10 minutes / Cooking time: 15 minutes

For soup:

4 cups spinach, chopped

1 cup green onion, chopped (green part only)

2 cups carrots, chopped

6 cups vegetable broth, low-FODMAP

1 tsp salt

For Meatballs:

1 lb ground pork

1 lb ground beef

1 tbsp gelatin

1 tbsp olive oil

¼ cup green onion, chopped (green part only)

2 tbsp fresh parsley, chopped

¼ tsp pepper

1 ½ tsp salt

- For meatballs: Preheat the oven to 350 F/ 180 C.
- Line baking tray with parchment paper and set aside.
- In a mixing bowl, combine together pork, beef, olive oil, green onion, parlay, pepper, salt, and gelatin.
- Make balls from meat mixture and place on a prepared baking tray and bake for 14 minutes.
- Meanwhile for soup: Add broth, green onion, carrots, and salt in a large stockpot and cook over medium heat until it starts to boiling then reduce heat to medium-low. Cover and cook for 10 minutes more.
- Add spinach and meatballs and cook for 5 minutes.
- Serve and enjoy.

Per Serving: Calories: 334; Total Fat: 11.2g; Saturated Fat: 3.4g; Protein: 48.9g; Carbs: 7g; Fiber: 1.9g; Sugar: 3.2g

Classic Antipasto Salad

Serves: 4 / Preparation time: 10 minutes / Cooking time: 5 minutes

For salad:

¼ cup fresh parsley, chopped

¼ cup capers, drained

8 oz cherry tomatoes, halved

½ cup green olives, sliced

½ cup black olives, sliced

1 cup bell pepper, chopped

½ cup sun-dried tomatoes, chopped

¼ cup artichoke hearts, drained and chopped

1 cup green onion, chopped (green part only)

For dressing:

1 tsp dried oregano

¼ cup red wine vinegar

¼ cup olive oil

¼ tsp pepper

¼ tsp salt

- In a large mixing bowl, add all salad ingredients and toss well.
- In a small bowl, whisk together all dressing ingredients.
- Pour dressing over salad.
- Toss well and serve.

Per Serving: Calories: 214; Total Fat: 17.7g; Saturated Fat: 2.6g; Protein: 2.9g; Carbs: 14.3g; Fiber: 3.8g; Sugar: 4.6g

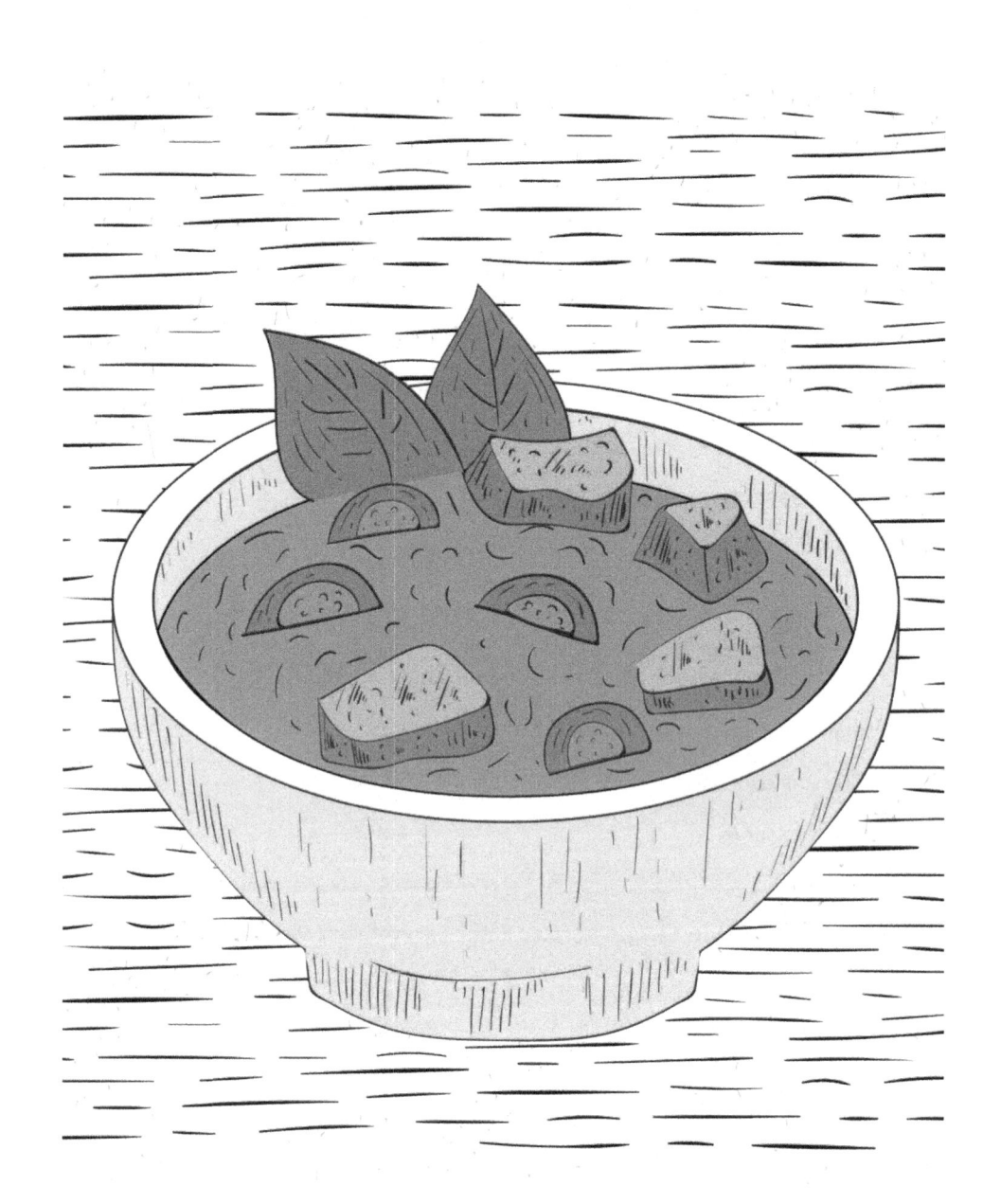

DINNER RECIPES

Contents

Pork Carnitas 86
Orange Chicken 87
Delicious Chicken Soup 88
Chicken Kabobs 89
Tasty Chicken Curry 90
Roasted Whole Turkey 91
Teriyaki Chicken 92
Tasty Cilantro Lime Chicken 93
Pesto Vegetable Chicken 94
Broiled Fish Fillets 95
Flavorful Rosemary Salmon 96
Tasty Pork Carnitas 97
Chicken & Rice 98
Perfect Baked Lemon Chicken 99
Simple Ranch Chicken 100
Simple Ranch Pork Chops 101
Pesto Zoodles 102
Tasty Ranch Potatoes 103
Easy Lemon Chicken 104
Flavorful Greek Chicken 105
Air Fryer Chicken Wings 106
Lemon Tomato Cod Fillets 107
Simple Turkey Breast 108
Delicious Pork Roast 109
Easy Pumpkin Soup 110
Ranch Pork Chops with Potatoes 111
Meatloaf 112
Djion Pork Chops 113
Salmon with Carrots 114
Perfect Moroccan Dinner 115

Pork Carnitas

Serves: 8 / Preparation time: 10 minutes / Cooking time: 8 hours 3 minutes

3 lbs pork roast

2 tbsp fresh cilantro, chopped

1 fresh lime juice

2 tbsp olive oil

- Place pork roast in a slow cooker.
- Cover and cook on low for 8 hours.
- Remove meat from slow cooker and shred using the fork.
- Heat oil in a large pan over medium-high heat.
- Add shredded meat to the pan and cook for 2-3 minutes.
- Remove from heat. Add lime juice and stir well.
- Garnish with cilantro and serve.

Per Serving: Calories: 384; Total Fat: 19.5g; Saturated Fat: 6.3g; Protein: 48.5g; Carbs: 0.5g; Fiber: 0g; Sugar: 0.1g

Orange Chicken

Serves: 6 / Preparation time: 10 minutes / Cooking time: 27 minutes

1 ½ lbs chicken thighs, skinless and boneless

1 tsp olive oil

½ tsp pepper

½ tsp ground coriander

1 tsp ground ginger

1 tsp salt

For sauce:

2 tbsp arrowroot powder

1 tbsp fish sauce

1 tbsp vinegar

¼ cup sunbutter

¼ cup coconut aminos

1 orange juice & zest

- Preheat the oven to 425 F/ 218 C.
- For the sauce: In a small bowl whisk together all sauce ingredients and set aside.
- For the chicken: In a large bowl, mix together coriander, ginger, pepper, and salt. Add chicken to the bowl and coat well with spice mixture.
- Heat oil in a large pan over medium-high heat.
- Add chicken to the pan and cook for 3-4 minutes. Turn chicken to other side and cook for 1 minute.
- Transfer chicken to a baking dish.
- Pour sauce mixture into the pan and cook until thickened, about 1-2 minutes.
- Pour sauce over chicken and bake the chicken in preheated oven for 15-20 minutes.
- Serve and enjoy.

Per Serving: Calories: 328; Total Fat: 14.6g; Saturated Fat: 3.1g; Protein: 35.6g; Carbs: 11.1g; Fiber: 2.2g; Sugar: 4g

Delicious Chicken Soup

Serves: 6 / Preparation time: 10 minutes / Cooking time: 30 minutes

For potato mixture:

1 lb potatoes, chopped

1 ½ cups unsweetened coconut milk

1 cup water

For soup:

2 lbs chicken, cooked and chopped

1 ½ cups green beans, chopped

1 tbsp fresh rosemary

1 tbsp fresh thyme

4 cups water

1 lb potatoes, diced

1 cup green onion, diced (green part only)

1 ½ cups carrots, chopped

2 tbsp olive oil

1 tsp salt

- In a small saucepan, mix together 1 cup of water and potatoes. Cover and cook for 10 minutes over medium heat. Once potatoes are cooked then drain well.
- Transfer potatoes in a large bowl along with coconut milk and blend using an immersion blender.
- Heat oil in a large pot. Add potatoes, green onion, and carrots and cook for 5 minutes.
- Add water, green beans, rosemary, thyme, and salt. Cover and cook for 10 minutes.
- Add chicken and potato puree to the pot. Stir well and cook for 10 minutes.
- Serve and enjoy.

Per Serving: Calories: 543; Total Fat: 23.9g; Saturated Fat: 14.8g; Protein: 49g; Carbs: 34.4g; Fiber: 7.8g; Sugar: 6.2g

Chicken Kabobs

Serves: 4 / Preparation time: 10 minutes / Cooking time: 10 minutes

1 ½ lbs chicken breast, skinless, boneless, and cut into 1-inch pieces

1 tbsp fresh lime juice

1 tbsp olive oil

1 tsp dried oregano

½ tsp pepper

½ tsp sea salt

- In a bowl, mix together lime juice, olive oil, oregano, pepper, and salt.
- Add chicken to the bowl and coat well with marinade. Cover and place in the refrigerator for overnight.
- Heat grill over medium heat.
- Remove chicken from refrigerator and thread it onto the soaked wooden skewers.
- Once the grill is hot then place chicken skewers onto the hot grill and cook for 8-10 minutes or until chicken is cooked.
- Serve hot and enjoy.

Per Serving: Calories: 226; Total Fat: 7.8g; Saturated Fat: 0.5g; Protein: 36.1g; Carbs: 0.5g; Fiber: 0.2g; Sugar: 0g

Tasty Chicken Curry

Serves: 4 / Preparation time: 10 minutes / Cooking time: 33 minutes

1 ½ lbs chicken thighs, skinless and boneless

1 tbsp olive oil

14 oz coconut milk

14 oz can roasted tomatoes, diced

1 tsp ground ginger

1 tbsp curry powder

1 tsp salt

- Add chicken in the instant pot. Add coconut milk, tomatoes, ginger, curry powder, oil, and salt over the chicken.
- Cover pot with a lid and select manual mode and set timer for 22 minutes.
- Once done then release pressure using the quick-release method than open the lid carefully.
- Remove chicken from pot. Set pot o sauté mode for 10 minutes.
- Cut chicken into the bite-size pieces and return into the instant pot.
- Stir well and serve.

Per Serving: Calories: 612; Total Fat: 40g; Saturated Fat: 25g; Protein: 52.5g; Carbs: 11.6g; Fiber: 4.4g; Sugar: 5.8g

Roasted Whole Turkey

Serves: 10 / Preparation time: 10 minutes / Cooking time: 2 hours 30 minutes

12 lbs whole turkey, remove giblets

2 tbsp fresh sage, chopped

2 tbsp fresh thyme, chopped

2 tbsp fresh rosemary, chopped

2 tsp olive oil

¾ cup ghee

1 tsp salt

- Preheat the oven to 350 F/ 180 C.
- Place turkey on a baking tray and pat dry with a paper towel.
- Tuck the turkey wings under the body and tie the turkey legs together with thick string.
- In a small bowl, mix together ghee, herbs, olive oil, and salt.
- Spread the ghee mixture all over the turkey.
- Bake turkey in preheated oven for 2 ½ hours or until the internal temperature of the turkey reaches to 160 F.
- Slice and serve.

Per Serving: Calories: 974; Total Fat: 55.3g; Saturated Fat: 21.9g; Protein: 102.2g; Carbs: 1g; Fiber: 0.6g; Sugar: 0g

Teriyaki Chicken

Serves: 6 / Preparation time: 10 minutes / Cooking time: 10 minutes

2 ½ lbs chicken thighs, skinless, boneless, and cut into small chunks

2 tsp cassava flour

1 tsp dried ginger

1 tbsp olive oil

1/3 cup water

2/3 cup coconut aminos

¼ cup orange juice

½ tsp salt

- In a small bowl, whisk together orange juice, cassava flour, ginger, oil, water, coconut aminos, and salt.
- Add chicken to the pan and pour orange juice mixture over the chicken.
- Cover and cook chicken over medium heat until cooked through, stir continuously 8-10 minutes.
- Serve and enjoy.

Per Serving: Calories: 411; Total Fat: 16.4g; Saturated Fat: 4.2g; Protein: 54.8g; Carbs: 6.6g; Fiber: 0.1g; Sugar: 0.9g

Tasty Cilantro Lime Chicken

Serves: 6 / Preparation time: 10 minutes / Cooking time: 10 minutes

1 ½ lbs chicken

4 tbsp fresh lime juice

2 tbsp olive oil

¾ cup fresh cilantro

1 tsp salt

- Add cilantro, lime juice, oil, and salt into the blender and blend until smooth.
- Place chicken in a large bowl then pours blended cilantro mixture over chicken and coat well. Cover and place in the refrigerator for 2 hours.
- Heat the grill over medium heat.
- Place marinated chicken onto the hot grill and cook for 5 minutes on each side or until chicken is cooked.
- Serve and enjoy.

Per Serving: Calories: 213; Total Fat: 8.1g; Saturated Fat: 1.6g; Protein: 32.9g; Carbs: 0.2g; Fiber: 0.1g; Sugar: 0g

Pesto Vegetable Chicken

Serves: 2/ Preparation time: 10 minutes / Cooking time: 7 hours

2 chicken breasts, skinless and boneless

2 cups zucchini, chopped

2 cups green beans, chopped

2 cups cherry tomatoes, halved

2 tbsp paleo pesto

- Place chicken breasts into the slow cooker.
- Pour pesto and vegetables over the chicken.
- Cover with lid and cook on low for 7 hours.
- Serve and enjoy.

Per Serving: Calories: 368; Total Fat: 15.6g; Saturated Fat: 3.7g; Protein: 39.3g; Carbs: 19.6g; Fiber: 7.4g; Sugar: 9.2g

Broiled Fish Fillets

Serves: 6 / Preparation time: 10 minutes / Cooking time: 5 minutes

24 oz tilapia fish fillets

1 tbsp olive oil

2 lemons, sliced

1/8 tsp cayenne pepper

¼ tsp cinnamon

½ tsp paprika

1 tsp dry mustard powder

½ tsp basil

½ tsp salt

- Line broiler pan with parchment paper and set aside.
- In a small bowl, mix together all dry spices.
- Place fish fillets on pan and brush with oil.
- Sprinkle spice mixture on fish fillets then arrange lemon slices on top of fish fillets.
- Broil fish fillets for 4-5 minutes.
- Serve and enjoy.

Per Serving: Calories: 280; Total Fat: 14.6g; Saturated Fat: 2.4g; Protein: 12.4g; Carbs: 25.3g; Fiber: 1.8g; Sugar: 1.5g

Flavorful Rosemary Salmon

Serves: 4 / Preparation time: 10 minutes / Cooking time: 15 minutes

1 ¼ lbs salmon, sliced into 4 pieces

1 tbsp dried chives

1 tbsp dried rosemary

1 tbsp olive oil

Pepper

Salt

- Preheat the oven to 425 F/ 218 C.
- Line baking tray with parchment paper and set aside.
- Place salmon pieces skin side down on the baking tray.
- Whisk together olive oil, chives, and rosemary and brush over salmon pieces.
- Bake salmon in preheated oven for 12-15 minutes. Season with pepper and salt.
- Serve and enjoy.

Per Serving: Calories: 221; Total Fat: 12.4g; Saturated Fat: 1.8g; Protein: 27.6g; Carbs: 0.6g; Fiber: 0.4g; Sugar: 0g

Tasty Pork Carnitas

Serves: 6 / Preparation time: 10 minutes / Cooking time: 9 Hours

3 lbs pork shoulder

2 tsp olive oil

2 tsp ground coriander

3 tsp cumin

2 orange juices

½ cup water

2 tsp salt

- Place the pork shoulder into the slow cooker.
- Pour remaining ingredients over the pork shoulder.
- Cover slow cooker with lid and cook on low for 9 hours.
- Remove meat from slow cooker and shred using a fork.
- Serve and enjoy.

Per Serving: Calories: 693; Total Fat: 50.4g; Saturated Fat: 18.1g; Protein: 53.2g; Carbs: 3.4g; Fiber: 0.2g; Sugar: 2.4g

Chicken & Rice

Serves: 4 / Preparation time: 10 minutes / Cooking time: 35 minutes

1 ½ lbs chicken breasts, skinless and boneless

2 cups spinach

2 cups water

1 cup white rice, uncooked

½ tsp turmeric

1 tbsp ginger, chopped

1 tomato, chopped

1 red bell pepper, chopped

1 tbsp olive oil

1 tsp paprika

1 tsp ground cumin

¼ tsp pepper

¼ tsp sea salt

- Season chicken with paprika, cumin, pepper, and salt.
- Heat oil in a large pan over medium-high heat.
- Add chicken to the pan and cook for 5-7 minutes on each side. Transfer chicken on a plate.
- Add ginger, tomato, and bell pepper to the pan and sauté for until soften.
- Add turmeric and stir for a minute.
- Add rice and water to the pan and stir well. Return chicken to the pan.
- Cover and cook over medium-low heat for 20 minutes or until all liquid is absorbed.
- Stir in spinach and cook until spinach is wilted.
- Serve and enjoy.

Per Serving: Calories: 547; Total Fat: 16.9g; Saturated Fat: 4.1g; Protein: 53.7g; Carbs: 42.1g; Fiber: 2g; Sugar: 2.2g

Perfect Baked Lemon Chicken

Serves: 4 / Preparation time: 10 minutes / Cooking time: 35 minutes

1 ¼ lbs chicken breasts, skinless and boneless

1 tbsp fresh parsley, chopped

2 tbsp fresh lemon juice

¼ cup water

3 tbsp butter, melted

1 tsp Italian seasoning

1 tbsp olive oil

Pepper

Salt

- Preheat the oven to 400 F/ 200 C.
- Season chicken with Italian seasoning, pepper, and salt.
- Heat oil in a large pan over medium-high heat.
- Add chicken to the pan and cook for 3-5 minutes on each side.
- Transfer chicken to a baking dish.
- In a small bowl, mix together butter, lemon juice, and water.
- Pour butter mixture over chicken and bake for 25 minutes.
- Garnish with parsley and serve.

Per Serving: Calories: 382; Total Fat: 23.1g; Saturated Fat: 9g; Protein: 41.2g; Carbs: 0.4g; Fiber: 0.1g; Sugar: 0.3g

Simple Ranch Chicken

Serves: 8 / Preparation time: 10 minutes / Cooking time: 10 minutes

2 lbs chicken breast, boneless and cut into chunks

2 tbsp olive oil

2 tbsp ranch seasoning, homemade

- Add chicken, ranch seasoning, and 1 tbsp oil in a bowl and toss well. Cover and place in the refrigerator for 15 minutes.
- Heat remaining oil in a pan over medium heat.
- Add chicken to the pan and cook for 4-5 minutes. Stir well and cook for 3-5 minutes more.
- Serve and enjoy.

Per Serving: Calories: 167; Total Fat: 6.3g; Saturated Fat: 0.5g; Protein: 24g; Carbs: 0g; Fiber: 0g; Sugar: 0g

Simple Ranch Pork Chops

Serves: 6 / Preparation time: 10 minutes / Cooking time: 35 minutes

6 pork chops, boneless

1 tsp dried parsley

2 tbsp ranch seasoning, homemade

¼ cup olive oil

Pepper

Salt

- Preheat the oven to 425 F/ 218 C.
- Season pork chops with pepper and salt and place on a baking tray.
- Mix together olive oil, parsley, and ranch seasoning.
- Spoon oil mixtures over pork chops and bake for 30 minutes.
- Broil pork chops for 5 minutes.
- Serve and enjoy.

Per Serving: Calories: 334; Total Fat: 28.3g; Saturated Fat: 8.7g; Protein: 18g; Carbs: 0g; Fiber: 0g; Sugar: 0g

Pesto Zoodles

Serves: 2 / Preparation time: 10 minutes / Cooking time: 5 minutes

2 zucchini, spiralized using a slicer

For pesto:

2 cups fresh spinach

2 tbsp olive oil

6 tbsp walnuts

1 tbsp fresh lemon juice

- Add all pesto ingredients into the blender and blend until smooth.
- Add zucchini noodles into the large mixing bowl.
- Pour pesto over zucchini noodles and toss well. Season with pepper and salt.
- Serve and enjoy.

Per Serving: Calories: 305; Total Fat: 28.3g; Saturated Fat: 2.9g; Protein: 8.9g; Carbs: 10.1g; Fiber: 4.4g; Sugar: 3.9g

Tasty Ranch Potatoes

Serves: 2 / Preparation time: 10 minutes / Cooking time: 10 minutes

1/2 lb potatoes, cut into 1-inch pieces

1/2 tbsp olive oil

1 tbsp ranch seasoning, homemade

- Preheat the air fryer at 375 F/ 190 C.
- Add all ingredients into the bowl and toss well.
- Transfer potato into the air fryer basket and cook for 10 minutes. Shake halfway through.
- Serve and enjoy.

Per Serving: Calories: 117; Total Fat: 3.6g; Saturated Fat: 0.5g; Protein: 1.9g; Carbs: 17.8g; Fiber: 2.7g; Sugar: 1.3g

Easy Lemon Chicken

Serves: 1 / Preparation time: 5 minutes / Cooking time: 15 minutes

1 chicken breast, boneless and skinless

1 fresh lemon, sliced

1/2 tbsp Italian seasoning

1 fresh lemon juice

Pepper

Salt

- Preheat the oven to 350 F/ 180 C.
- Season chicken with Italian season, pepper and salt.
- Place chicken breast onto the foil piece. Pour lemon juice over chicken and arrange lemon slices on top of chicken.
- Tightly fold foil around the chicken breast and place in air fryer basket and cook for 15 minutes.
- Serve and enjoy.

Per Serving: Calories: 179; Total Fat: 5.5g; Saturated Fat: 0.7g; Protein: 25.1g; Carbs: 7.2g; Fiber: 1.8g; Sugar: 3.1g

Flavorful Greek Chicken

Serves: 6 / Preparation time: 10 minutes / Cooking time: 10 minutes

2 lbs chicken thighs, skinless and boneless

1/2 cup olives

1/2 tsp ground coriander

3/4 tsp chili pepper

1/2 tsp paprika

2 tbsp olive oil

28 oz can tomato, diced

2 tsp dried oregano

2 tsp dried parsley

Pepper

Salt

- Add oil in the instant pot and set the pot on sauté mode.
- Add chicken to the pot and sauté until brown. Transfer chicken on a plate.
- Add tomatoes, spices, pepper, and salt and cook for 2-3 minutes.
- Return chicken to the pot and stir well to combine.
- Seal pot with lid and cook on manual mode for 8 minutes.
- Once done then release pressure using quick-release method than open the lid.
- Add olives and stir well.
- Serve and enjoy.

Per Serving: Calories: 275; Total Fat: 12.9g; Saturated Fat: 2.9g; Protein: 33.7g; Carbs: 4.5g; Fiber: 1.2g; Sugar: 2.2g

Air Fryer Chicken Wings

Serves: 4 / Preparation time: 10 minutes / Cooking time: 16 minutes

1 lb chicken wings

1 tbsp olive oil

1 tsp lemon pepper seasoning

1 tsp salt

- Add chicken wings, oil, lemon pepper seasoning, and salt into the large bowl and toss well.
- Place chicken wings in the air fryer basket and cook at 400 F/ 200 C for 8 minutes.
- Turn chicken wings to other side and cook for 8 minutes more.
- Serve and enjoy.

Per Serving: Calories: 247; Total Fat: 11.9g; Saturated Fat: 2.8g; Protein: 32.9g; Carbs: 0.3g; Fiber: 0.1g; Sugar: 0g

Lemon Tomato Cod Fillets

Serves: 6 / Preparation time: 10 minutes / Cooking time: 5 minutes

1 1/2 lb cod fillets

1 tsp oregano

1 lemon juice

28 oz can tomatoes, diced

3 tbsp olive oil

1/2 tsp pepper

1 tsp salt

- Add olive oil into the instant pot and set the pot on sauté mode.
- Add tomatoes, lemon juice, oregano, pepper, and salt and stir for 2 minutes.
- Add fish fillets and stir well.
- Seal pot with lid and cook on high pressure for 3 minutes.
- Once done then release pressure using quick-release method than open the lid.
- Serve and enjoy.

Per Serving: Calories: 182; Total Fat: 8.1g; Saturated Fat: 1.1g; Protein: 21.6g; Carbs: 7.2g; Fiber: 2.4g; Sugar: 4.7g

Simple Turkey Breast

Serves: 12 / Preparation time: 10 minutes / Cooking time: 4 hours

6 lbs turkey breast, bone-in

1/2 cup water

4 fresh rosemary sprigs

Pepper

Salt

- Season turkey breast with pepper and salt and place in the slow cooker.
- Add water and rosemary on top.
- Cover with lid and cook on low for 4 hours.
- Serve and enjoy.

Per Serving: Calories: 236; Total Fat: 3.8g; Saturated Fat: 0.8g; Protein: 38.7g; Carbs: 9.6g; Fiber: 1.1g; Sugar: 8g

Delicious Pork Roast

Serves: 6 / Preparation time: 10 minutes / Cooking time: 8 hours

3 lbs pork shoulder roast, boneless and cut into 4 pieces

2/3 cup grapefruit juice

1/2 tbsp cumin

1 tbsp fresh oregano

Pepper

Salt

- Season meat with pepper and salt and place into the slow cooker.
- Add cumin, oregano, and grapefruit juice into the blender and blend until smooth.
- Pour blended mixture over meat and stir well.
- Cover with lid and cook on low for 8 hours.
- Remove meat from slow cooker and shred using a fork.
- Return shredded meat into the slow cooker and stir well.
- Serve and enjoy.

Per Serving: Calories: 594; Total Fat: 46.4g; Saturated Fat: 16.1g; Protein: 38.4g; Carbs: 2.7g; Fiber: 0.6g; Sugar: 1.8g

Easy Pumpkin Soup

Serves: 4 / Preparation time: 10 minutes / Cooking time: 8 hours

2 cups pumpkin puree

1 cup coconut milk

4 cups water

1/4 tsp ground nutmeg

- Add all ingredients into the slow cooker and stir well.
- Cover with lid and cook on low for 8 hours.
- Puree the soup using an immersion blender until smooth.
- Stir well and serve.

Per Serving: Calories: 180; Total Fat: 14.7g; Saturated Fat: 12.9g; Protein: 2.7g; Carbs: 13.3g; Fiber: 4.9g; Sugar: 6.1g

Ranch Pork Chops with Potatoes

Serves: 4 / Preparation time: 10 minutes / Cooking time: 35 minutes

4 pork chops, boneless

¼ tsp ground oregano

1 tsp dried parsley

3 tbsp olive oil

1 oz ranch seasoning, homemade

2 ½ lbs potatoes, cut into bite-size pieces

¼ tsp pepper

- Preheat the oven to 400 F/ 200 C.
- Spray a baking tray with cooking spray and set aside.
- In a small bowl, mix together ranch seasoning mix, oregano, parsley, oil, and pepper.
- Add potatoes and 1 ½ tbsp seasoning mixture to the bowl and toss well.
- Place potatoes on a baking tray and cook for 20 minutes.
- Season pork chops with remaining seasoning. Set potatoes one side of the baking tray and arrange pork chops on a baking tray.
- Bake pork chops for 10-15 minutes.
- Serve and enjoy.

Per Serving: Calories: 542; Total Fat: 30.7g; Saturated Fat: 9g; Protein: 22.8g; Carbs: 44.7g; Fiber: 6.9g; Sugar: 3.3g

Meatloaf

Serves: 6 / Preparation time: 10 minutes / Cooking time: 55 minutes

2 lbs ground beef	½ cup sunflower seed flour
1 tsp oregano	½ cup salsa, low-fodmap
1 tsp paprika	2 eggs, lightly beaten
1 tsp cumin	2 tbsp olive oil
1.4 cup fresh cilantro, chopped	1 red bell pepper, diced
¼ cup green onion, chopped (green part only)	½ tsp salt

- Preheat the oven to 375 F/ 190 C.
- Spray a loaf pan with cooking spray and set aside.
- Add meat in a bowl. Cook bell pepper in olive oil over medium heat, about 5 minutes.
- Transfer bell pepper in meat bowl.
- Add remaining ingredients to the meat mixture and mix until well combined.
- Transfer meat mixture into the loaf pan and bake in preheated oven for 50-55 minutes.
- Slice and serve.

Per Serving: Calories: 377; Total Fat: 15.9g; Saturated Fat: 4.7g; Protein: 51.1g; Carbs: 5.8g; Fiber: 1.4g; Sugar: 2g

Djion Pork Chops

Serves: 4 / Preparation time: 10 minutes / Cooking time: 10 minutes

4 pork chops, boneless

2 tbsp fresh rosemary, chopped

¼ cup coconut aminos

2 tbsp olive oil

¼ cup Dijon mustard

½ tsp salt

- In a bowl, mix together rosemary, coconut aminos, olive oil, Dijon mustard, and salt.
- Add pork chops to the bowl and coat well. Cover and place in the refrigerator for 1 hour.
- Heat grill over medium-high heat.
- Place marinated pork chops onto the hot grill and cook for 5 minutes on each side.
- Serve and enjoy.

Per Serving: Calories: 347; Total Fat: 27.8g; Saturated Fat: 8.6g; Protein: 18.7g; Carbs: 4.9g; Fiber: 1.2g; Sugar: 0.1g

Salmon with Carrots

Serves: 4 / Preparation time: 10 minutes / Cooking time: 20 minutes

1 lb salmon, cut into four pieces

2 cups baby carrots

2 tbsp olive oil

Salt

- Preheat the oven to 425 F/ 218 C.
- Place salmon pieces on the center of the baking tray.
- In a mixing bowl, toss together baby carrots and olive oil.
- Arrange carrot around the salmon and bake in preheated oven for 20 minutes.
- Season salmon and carrots with salt.
- Serve and enjoy.

Per Serving: Calories: 210; Total Fat: 14g; Saturated Fat: 2g; Protein: 22g; Carbs: 4g; Fiber: 1.5g; Sugar: 2.5g

Perfect Moroccan Dinner

Serves: 4 / Preparation time: 10 minutes / Cooking time: 25 minutes

1 lb chicken breasts, cut into pieces

2 tbsp olive oil

1 tbsp fresh lemon juice

1 tsp turmeric

2 tsp ginger, minced

1 ½ tbsp dried chives

1 tbsp dried parsley

1 tbsp fresh mint, chopped

1 small eggplant, cubed

1 sweet potato, cubed

6 carrots, chopped

¼ tsp pepper

1 tsp sea salt

- Preheat the oven to 400 F/ 200 C.
- Add all ingredients into the large mixing bowl and toss to coat.
- Transfer vegetable and chicken mixture onto the baking tray and bake for 25-30 minutes or until the internal temperature of chicken reaches to 165 F.
- Serve and enjoy.

Per Serving: Calories: 375; Total Fat: 15.8g; Saturated Fat: 3.4g; Protein: 35.5g; Carbs: 23g; Fiber: 7.7g; Sugar: 10g

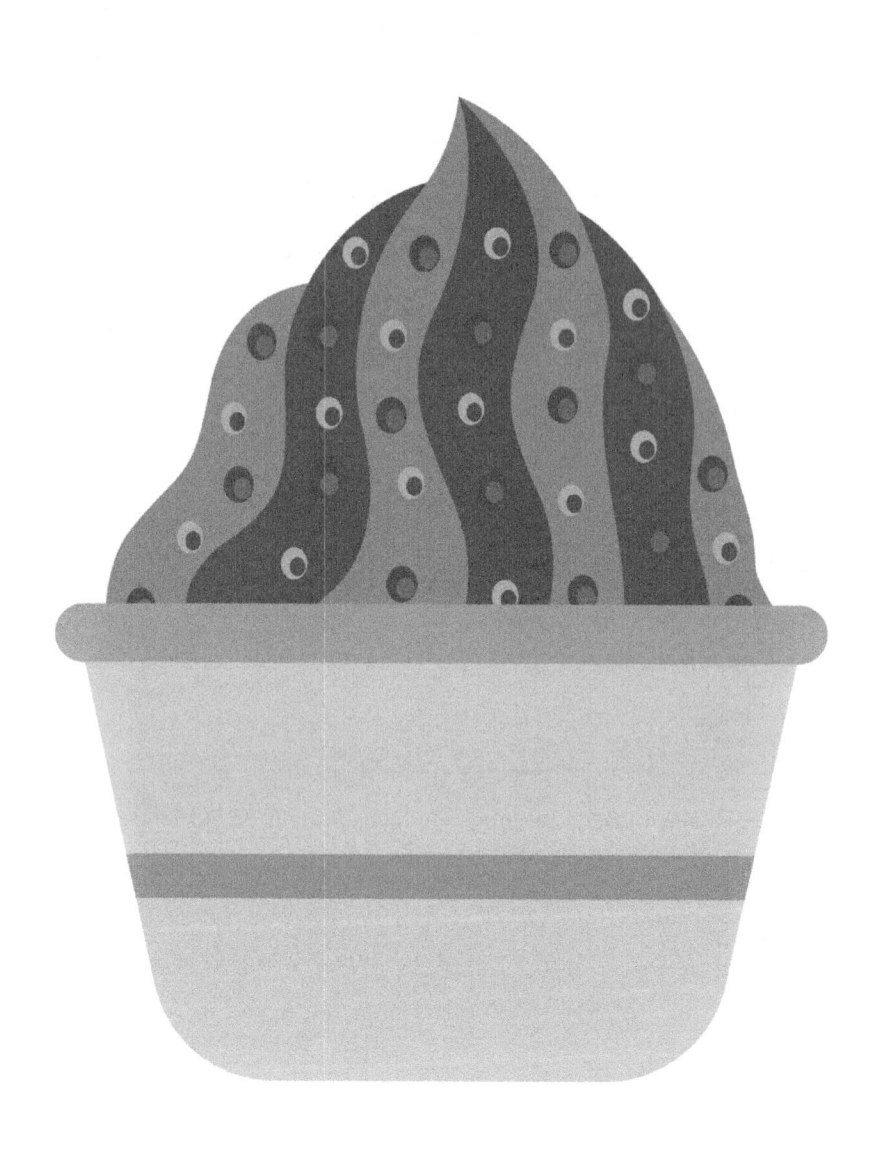

DESSERT RECIPES

Contents

Refreshing Mojito Popsicles 118
Chia Strawberry Popsicles 119
Blueberry Sorbet 120
Strawberry Sorbet 121
Strawberry Gummies 122
Chocolate Fudge 123
Easy Lemon Curd 124
Nut-Free Brownies 125
Canteloupe Popsicles 126
Skillet Brownie 127

Refreshing Mojito Popsicles

Serves: 4 / Preparation time: 5 minutes / Cooking time: 5 minutes

2 cups water

¼ cup fresh mint, chopped

1 lime juice

1 lime zest

- Mix together water, mint, lime zest, and lime juice.
- Pour mixture into the Popsicle molds and place in the refrigerator for overnight.
- Serve and enjoy.

Per Serving: Calories: 5; Total Fat: 0.1g; Saturated Fat: 0g; Protein: 0.2g; Carbs: 1.4g; Fiber: 0.4g; Sugar: 0.2g

Chia Strawberry Popsicles

Serves: 4 / Preparation time: 5 minutes / Cooking time: 5 minutes

½ cup strawberries

2 tsp chia seeds

1 tbsp fresh lemon juice

½ cup water

- Add all ingredients into the blender and blend until smooth.
- Pour blended mixture into the Popsicle molds and place in refrigerator until set.
- Serve and enjoy.

Per Serving: Calories: 12; Total Fat: 0.5g; Saturated Fat: 0.1g; Protein: 0.4g; Carbs: 1.7g; Fiber: 0.4g; Sugar: 1g

Blueberry Sorbet

Serves: 1 / Preparation time: 5 minutes / Cooking time: 5 minutes

7 oz frozen blueberries

1 tbsp fresh lemon juice

1 tsp maple syrup

- Add all ingredients into the blender and blend until smooth.
- Pour blended mixture into the air-tight container and place in refrigerator until firm.
- Serve chilled and enjoy.

Per Serving: Calories: 135; Total Fat: 0.8g; Saturated Fat: 0.1g; Protein: 1.6g; Carbs: 33.5g; Fiber: 4.9g; Sugar: 24g

Strawberry Sorbet

Serves: 4 / Preparation time: 5 minutes / Cooking time: 5 minutes

16 oz frozen strawberries, halved   ¼ cup maple syrup

- Add all ingredients into the blender and blend until smooth.
- Pour blended mixture into the air-tight container and place in refrigerator until firm.
- Serve chilled and enjoy.

Per Serving: Calories: 88; Total Fat: 0.4g; Saturated Fat: 0g; Protein: 0.8g; Carbs: 21.9g; Fiber: 2.3g; Sugar: 17.3g

Strawberry Gummies

Serves: 12 / Preparation time: 10 minutes / Cooking time: 20 minutes

1 cup strawberries, chopped

3 tbsp maple syrup

¼ cup water

¼ cup gelatin

2/3 cup fresh lemon juice

- Add strawberries, water, and lemon juice into the blender and blend until pureed.
- Pour blended mixture into the pan and heat over medium-low heat.
- Slowly add gelatin and stir until gelatin is dissolved.
- Once the gelatin is completely dissolved then stir in maple syrup.
- Remove pan from heat and let it cool for 5 minutes.
- Pour gelatin mixture into the candy mold and place in the refrigerator for 2 hours or until set.
- Serve and enjoy.

Per Serving: Calories: 34; Total Fat: 0.2g; Saturated Fat: 0.1g; Protein: 0.5g; Carbs: 7.7g; Fiber: 0.3g; Sugar: 6.9g

Chocolate Fudge

Serves: 10 / Preparation time: 10 minutes / Cooking time: 10 minutes

½ cup cashew butter ½ cup coconut oil
½ cup unsweetened chocolate chips

- Line 9*5-inch loaf pan with parchment paper and set aside.
- Add all ingredients into the double boiler on medium heat until melted. Stir well.
- Pour melted mixture into the prepared pan and place in refrigerator until set.
- Cut into pieces and serve.

Per Serving: Calories: 249; Total Fat: 23.6g; Saturated Fat: 14.7g; Protein: 3.9g; Carbs: 6.7g; Fiber: 1.9g; Sugar: 0.6g

Easy Lemon Curd

Serves: 6 / Preparation time: 10 minutes / Cooking time: 5 minutes

3 eggs, lightly beaten

¼ cup ghee

½ cup fresh lemon juice

1 tbsp lemon zest

5 tbsp maple syrup

Pinch of salt

- Add eggs, lemon juice, lemon zest, maple syrup, and salt in a pan and whisk well to combine.
- Cook pan mixture over medium heat and stir constantly for 5 minutes.
- Remove from heat and add ghee and whisk well.
- Strain mixture through a strainer over a bowl.
- Store in the fridge and serve.

Per Serving: Calories: 155; Total Fat: 10.9g; Saturated Fat: 6.1g; Protein: 3g; Carbs: 12g; Fiber: 0.1g; Sugar: 10.6g

Nut-Free Brownies

Serves: 6 / Preparation time: 10 minutes / Cooking time: 20 minutes

2 eggs, lightly beaten

1 medium zucchini, shredded and squeeze out all liquid

¼ cup coconut flour

½ cup unsweetened cocoa powder

¼ cup unsweetened coconut milk

¼ cup maple syrup

1 cup sunbutter

- Preheat the oven to 350 F/ 180 C.
- Line 8*8-inch baking dish with parchment paper and set aside.
- In a large bowl, combine together sunbutter, milk, eggs, and maple syrup.
- Add coconut flour, zucchini, and cocoa powder and stir to combine.
- Transfer batter in a prepared baking dish and bake for 20 minutes.
- Slice and serve.

Per Serving: Calories: 369; Total Fat: 26.3g; Saturated Fat: 5.9g; Protein: 13.3g; Carbs: 24.1g; Fiber: 8.5g; Sugar: 13g

Canteloupe Popsicles

Serves: 10 / Preparation time: 10 minutes / Cooking time: 5 minutes

4 ½ cups cantaloupe, chopped

14 oz can coconut milk, full-fat

- Add all ingredients into the blender and blend until smooth.
- Pour blended mixture into the popsicle molds and place in the refrigerator for overnight.
- Serve and enjoy.

Per Serving: Calories: 50; Total Fat: 2.5g; Saturated Fat: 2g; Protein: 1.3g; Carbs: 6.4g; Fiber: 0.6g; Sugar: 6.2g

Skillet Brownie

Serves: 2 / Preparation time: 10 minutes / Cooking time: 10 minutes

2 tbsp coconut flour
2 tbsp unsweetened cocoa powder
1 egg, lightly beaten
½ tsp vanilla

¼ cup maple syrup
½ cup sunbutter
¼ tsp salt

- Preheat the oven to 350 F/ 180 C.
- Spray two 6.5-inch skillets with cooking spray and set aside.
- In a bowl, combine together sunbutter, egg, vanilla, maple syrup, and salt.
- Add coconut flour and cocoa powder and stir to combine.
- Divide brownie mixture evenly between two skillets and bake in preheated oven for 10 minutes.
- Serve and enjoy.

Per Serving: Calories: 616; Total Fat: 37g; Saturated Fat: 5.1g; Protein: 21.8g; Carbs: 51.7g; Fiber: 12.8g; Sugar: 32.8g

REFERENCES AND RESOURCES

Aboutibs.org. (2017). *Five Low FODMAP Diet Pitfalls (and What You Can Do to Avoid Them)*. [online] Available at: https://aboutibs.org/low-fodmap-diet/five-low-fodmap-diet-pitfalls-and-what-you-can-do-to-avoid-them

Ballantyne, S. (2014). *The Paleo Approach*. 1st ed. Victory Belt Publishing.

Barrett, J. (2017). How to institute the low-FODMAP diet. *Journal of Gastroenterology and Hepatology*, 32, pp.8-10.

Boers, Inge, et al. "Favourable Effects of Consuming a Palaeolithic-Type Diet on Characteristics of the Metabolic Syndrome: a Randomized Controlled Pilot-Study." *Lipids in Health and Disease*, BioMed Central, 11 Oct. 2014, lipidworld.biomedcentral.com/articles/10.1186/1476-511X-13-160.

Chey, W. and Whelan, K. (2016). Dietary guidelines for irritable bowel syndrome are important for gastroenterologists, dietitians and people with irritable bowel syndrome. *Journal of Human Nutrition and Dietetics*, 29(5), pp.547-548.

Cordain L. The nutritional characteristics of a contemporary diet based upon Paleolithic food groups. Journal of the American Nutraceutical Association. 2002;5(3):15-24.

Gearry, R., Skidmore, P., O'Brien, L., Wilkinson, T. and Nanayakkara, W. (2016). Efficacy of the low FODMAP diet for treating irritable bowel syndrome: the evidence to date. *Clinical and Experimental Gastroenterology*, p.131.

Hoffman R. Can the paleolithic diet meet the nutritional needs of older people? Maturitas. 2017;95:63-64. doi:10.1016/j.maturitas.2016.09.005.

H. Shmerling, R. (2018). *Autoimmune disease and stress: Is there a link? - Harvard Health Blog*. [online] Harvard Health Blog. Available at: https://www.health.harvard.edu/blog/autoimmune-disease-and-stress-is-there-a-link-2018071114230

Indumathy, P. and Ramya, J. (2018). Impact of Lifestyle Modifications and Paleo Diet on Selected Obese Subjects. *FoodSci: Indian Journal of Research in Food Science and Nutrition*, 5(2), p.44.

Manheimer, E., van Zuuren, E., Fedorowicz, Z. and Pijl, H. (2015). Paleolithic nutrition for metabolic syndrome: systematic review and meta-analysis. *The American Journal of Clinical Nutrition*, 102(4), pp.922-932.

Mellberg, C., Sandberg, S., Ryberg, M., Eriksson, M., Brage, S., Larsson, C., Olsson, T. and Lindahl, B. (2014). Long-term effects of a Palaeolithic-type diet in obese postmenopausal women: a 2-year randomized trial. *European Journal of Clinical Nutrition*, 68(3), pp.350-357.

Monashfodmap.com. (n.d.). *Starting the Low FODMAP Diet | Monash FODMAP Monash Fodmap*. [online] Available at: https://www.monashfodmap.com/ibs-central/i-have-ibs/starting-the-low-fodmap-diet/

Obert J, Pearlman M, Obert L, Chapin S. Popular weight loss strategies: a review of four weight loss techniques. *Current gastroenterology reports*. 2017 Dec 1;19(12):61.

Österdahl M, Kocturk T, Koochek A, Wändell PE. Effects of a short-term intervention with a paleolithic diet in healthy volunteers. *European journal of clinical nutrition*. 2008 May;62(5):682.

Shepherd, S. and Gibson, P. (2013). *The Complete Low FODMAP Diet*. New York: The Experiment.

Staudacher, H. (2017). Nutritional, microbiological and psychosocial implications of the low FODMAP diet. *Journal of Gastroenterology and Hepatology*, 32, pp.16-19.

Stewart, L., D. M. Edgar, J., Blakely, G. and Patrick, S. (2018). Antigenic mimicry of ubiquitin by the gut bacterium Bacteroides fragilis: a potential link with autoimmune disease. *Clinical & Experimental Immunology*, 194(2), pp.153-165.

UC Davis Health, D. (2015). *Is the paleo diet safe for your health? | UC Davis Health*. [online] Health.ucdavis.edu. Available at: https://health.ucdavis.edu/welcome/features/2014-2015/06/20150603_paleo-diet.html

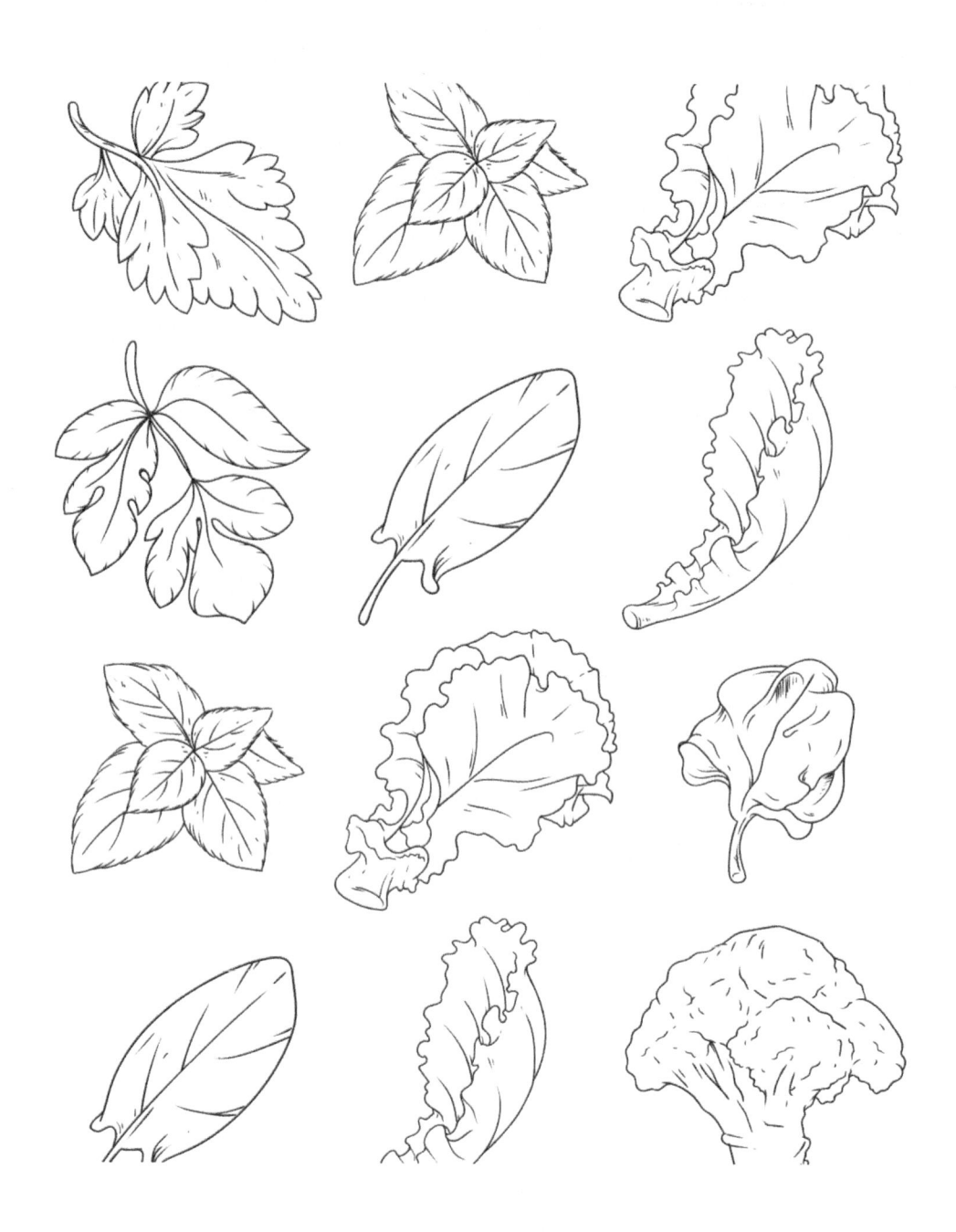

THE "DIRTY DOZEN" AND "CLEAN 15"

Every year, the Environmental Working Group releases a list of the produce with the most pesticide residue (Dirty Dozen) and a list of the ones with the least chance of having residue (Clean 15). It's based on analysis from the U.S. Department of Agriculture Pesticide Data Program report.

The Environmental Working Group found that 70% of the 48 types of produce tested had residues of at least one type of pesticide. In total there were 178 different pesticides and pesticide breakdown products. This residue can stay on veggies and fruit even after they are washed and peeled. All pesticides are toxic to humans and consuming them can cause damage to the nervous system, reproductive system, cancer, a weakened immune system, and more. Women who are pregnant can expose their unborn children to toxins through their diet, and continued exposure to pesticides can affect their development.

This info can help you choose the best fruits and veggies, as well as which ones you should always try to buy organic.

The Dirty Dozen

- Strawberries
- Spinach
- Nectarines
- Apples
- Peaches
- Celery
- Grapes
- Pears
- Cherries
- Tomatoes
- Sweet bell peppers
- Potatoes

The Clean 15

- Sweet corn
- Avocados
- Pineapples
- Cabbage
- Onions
- Frozen sweet peas
- Papayas
- Asparagus
- Mangoes
- Eggplant
- Honeydew
- Kiwi
- Cantaloupe
- Cauliflower
- Grapefruit

132 THE "DIRTY DOZEN" AND "CLEAN 15"

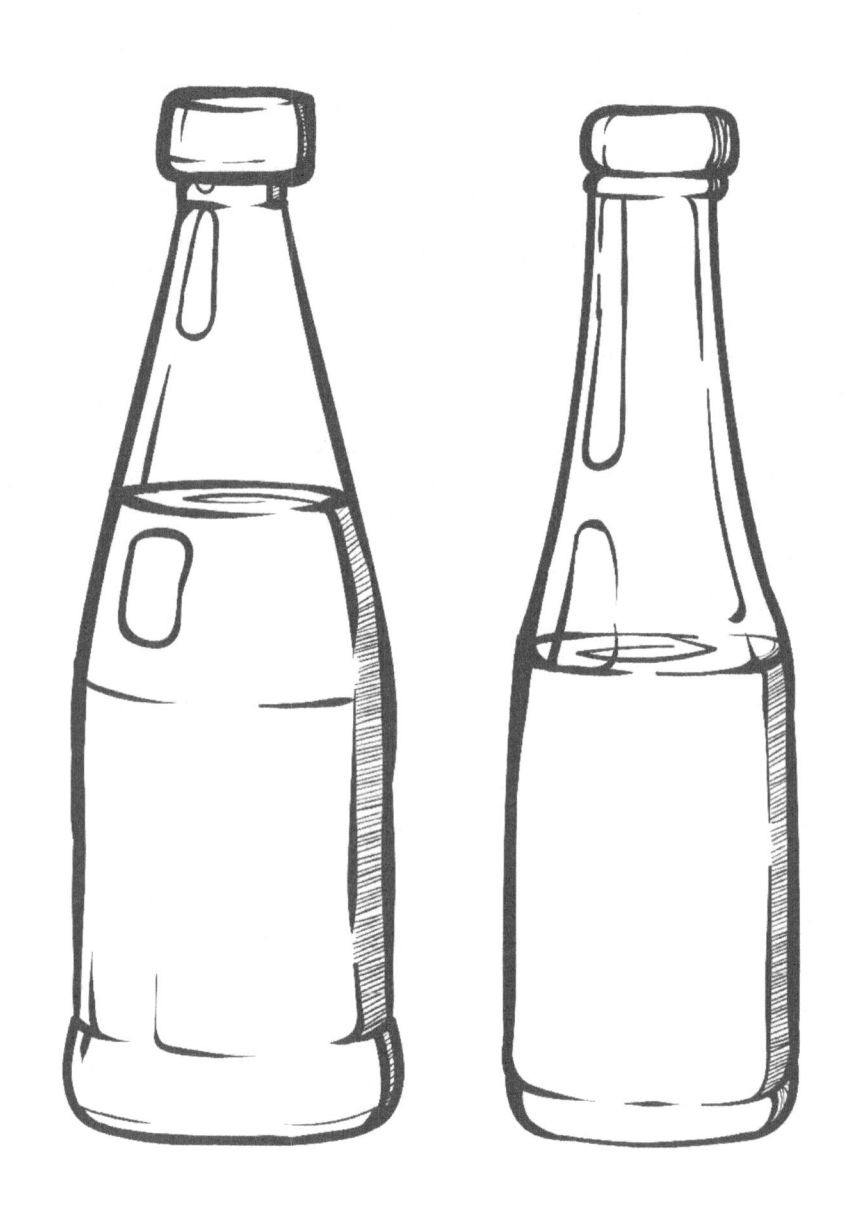

MEASUREMENT CONVERSION TABLES

Volume Equivalents (Dry)

US Standard	Metric (Approx.)
¼ teaspoon	1 ml
½ teaspoon	2 ml
1 teaspoon	5 ml
1 tablespoon	15 ml
¼ cup	59 ml
½ cup	118 ml
1 cup	235 ml

Weight Equivalents

US Standard	Metric (Approx.)
½ ounce	15 g
1 ounce	30 g
2 ounces	60 g
4 ounces	115 g
8 ounces	225 g
12 ounces	340 g
16 oz or 1 lb	455 g

Volume Equivalents (Liquid)

US Standard	US Standard (ounces)	Metric (Approx.)
2 tablespoons	1 fl oz	30 ml
¼ cup	2 fl oz	60 ml
½ cup	4 fl oz	120 ml
1 cup	8 fl oz	240 ml
1 ½ cups	12 fl oz	355 ml
2 cups or 1 pint	16 fl oz	475 ml
4 cups or 1 quart	32 fl oz	1 L
1 gallon	128 fl oz	4 L

Oven Temperatures

Fahrenheit (F)	Celsius (C) (Approx)
250°F	120°C
300°F	150°C
325°F	165°C
350°F	180°C
375°F	190°C
400°F	200°C
425°F	220°C
450°F	230°C

INDEX

A
Air Fryer Chicken Wings, 106

B
Banana Strawberry Smoothie, 48
Blueberry Sorbet, 120
Breakfast Egg Muffins, 39
Broiled Fish Fillets, 95

C
Canteloupe Popsicles, 126
Chia Strawberry Popsicles, 119
Chicken & Rice, 98
Chicken Berry Salad, 56
Chicken Chili, 66
Chicken Chili Soup, 67
Chicken Egg Muffins, 43
Chicken Kabobs, 89
Chicken Zoodle Soup, 68
Choco Chia Pudding, 37
Chocolate Fudge, 123
Classic Antipasto Salad, 83
Coconut Fish Stew, 71
Cucumber Tomato Salad, 69
Curried Chicken Soup, 70

D
Delicious Breakfast Bake, 23
Delicious Chicken Green Chile, 73
Delicious Chicken Soup, 88
Delicious Pepper Soup, 63
Delicious Pork Roast, 109
Delicious Pumpkin Scones, 51
Djion Pork Chops, 113

E
Easy Braised Turnips, 81
Easy Egg Salad, 79
Easy Lemon Chicken, 104
Easy Lemon Curd, 124
Easy Pesto Chicken Salad, 64
Easy Pumpkin Soup, 110
Egg Bacon Muffins, 40
Egg Scramble, 35

F
Flavorful Chicken Salad, 54
Flavorful Greek Chicken, 105
Flavorful Rosemary Salmon, 96
Flavors Picadillo, 61

G
Greek Chicken Salad, 55
Green Beans with Pine Nuts, 78
Green Tropical Smoothie, 49

H
Healthy Breakfast Frittata, 31
Healthy Kale Salad, 74
Herb Zucchini Noodles, 76

I
Italian Breakfast Sausage, 26
Italian Meatball Soup, 82

K
Kale Pineapple Smoothie, 30
Kiwi Green Smoothie, 33

L
Lemon Chicken Salad, 77
Lemon Tomato Cod Fillets, 107

M
Mashed Potatoes, 28
Meat Patties, 65
Meatloaf, 112
Mint Pineapple Smoothie, 34

N

Nut-Free Brownies, 125

O

Orange Chicken, 87

P

Perfect Baked Lemon Chicken, 99
Perfect Moroccan Dinner, 115
Pesto Vegetable Chicken, 94
Pesto Zoodles, 102
Pork Carnitas, 86
Potato Salad, 57
Pulled Pork, 59
Pumpkin Smoothie, 45

R

Ranch Pork Chops with Potatoes, 111
Refreshing Kiwi Green Smoothie, 47
Refreshing Mojito Popsicles, 118
Roasted Veggies, 80
Roasted Whole Turkey, 91

S

Salmon Cakes, 36
Salmon Waffles, 29
Salmon with Carrots, 114
Sausage Kale Egg Muffins, 44
Sauteed Shrimp, 38
Simple Ranch Chicken, 100
Simple Ranch Pork Chops, 101
Simple Turkey Breast, 108
Skillet Brownie, 127
Spinach Basil Egg Scramble, 46
Spinach Berry Smoothie, 32
Spinach Pepper Egg Bites, 41
Spinach Pepper Frittata, 25
Strawberry Gummies, 122
Strawberry kale Salad, 75
Strawberry Sorbet, 121
Summer Veggie Soup, 72

T

Tasty Chicken Curry, 90
Tasty Cilantro Lime Chicken, 93
Tasty Crab Cake Waffles, 27
Tasty Pork Carnitas, 97
Tasty Ranch Potatoes, 103
Teriyaki Chicken, 92
Tomato Chicken Soup, 58
Tuna Waffles, 50
Turkey Meatballs, 60
Turnip Dill Puree, 24

Z

Zucchini Chicken Meatballs, 62
Zucchini Egg Muffins, 42
Zucchini Sausage Casserole, 22

Made in the USA
Monee, IL
28 December 2021